Practical TIPS For BACK SURGERY

Practical TIPS For BACK SURGERY

From Preparation to Recovery
(or How to Get Your Undies On When You Can't Reach Your Feet!)

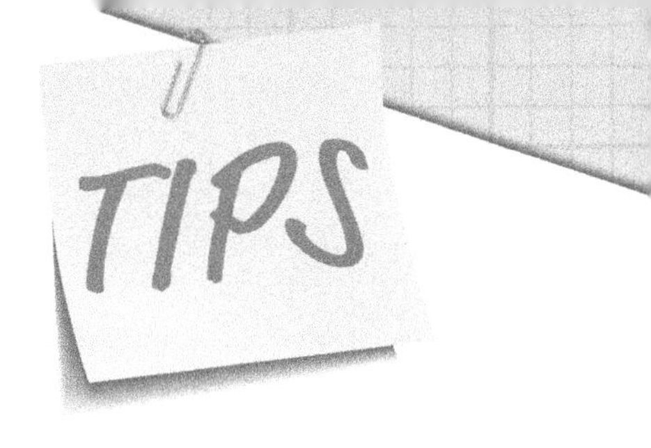

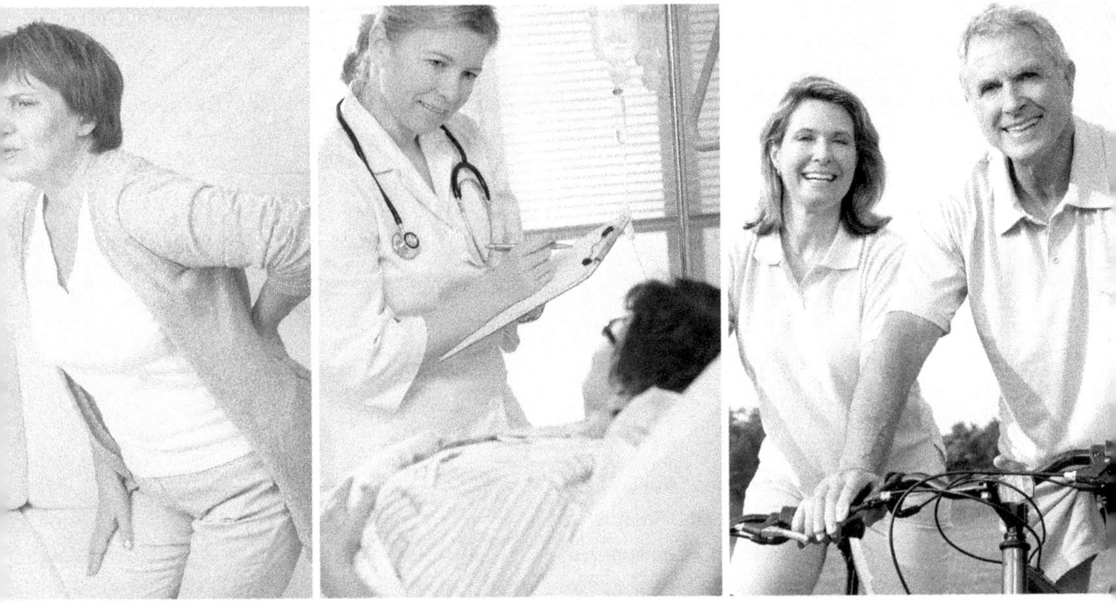

JACKIE TALLENTYRE

DISCLAIMER

All the information, techniques, skills and concepts contained within this publication are of the nature of general comment only and are not in any way recommended as individual advice. The intent is to offer a variety of information to provide a wider range of choices now and in the future, recognising that we all have widely diverse circumstances and viewpoints. Should any reader choose to make use of the information contained herein, this is their decision, and the contributors (and their companies), authors and publishers do not assume any responsibilities whatsoever under any condition or circumstances. It is recommended that the reader obtain their own independent advice.

First Edition 2017

National Library of Australia

Cataloguing-in-Publication entry:

Creator: Tallentyre, Jackie, 1964- author.

Title: Practical Tips For Back Surgery : From Preparation to Recovery (Or How to Get Your Undies On When You Can't Reach Your Feet!) / Jackie Tallentyre.

ISBN: 9781925288391 (paperback)

Subjects: Back--Surgery--Rehabilitation--Popular works.
Backache--Treatment--Popular works.
Backache--Physical therapy--Popular works.
Pain--Treatment--Popular works.

Dewey Number: 617.564

Published by Global Publishing Group
PO Box 517 Mt Evelyn, Victoria 3796 Australia
Email info@GlobalPublishingGroup.com.au

For further information about orders:
Phone: +61 3 9739 4686 or Fax +61 3 8648 6871

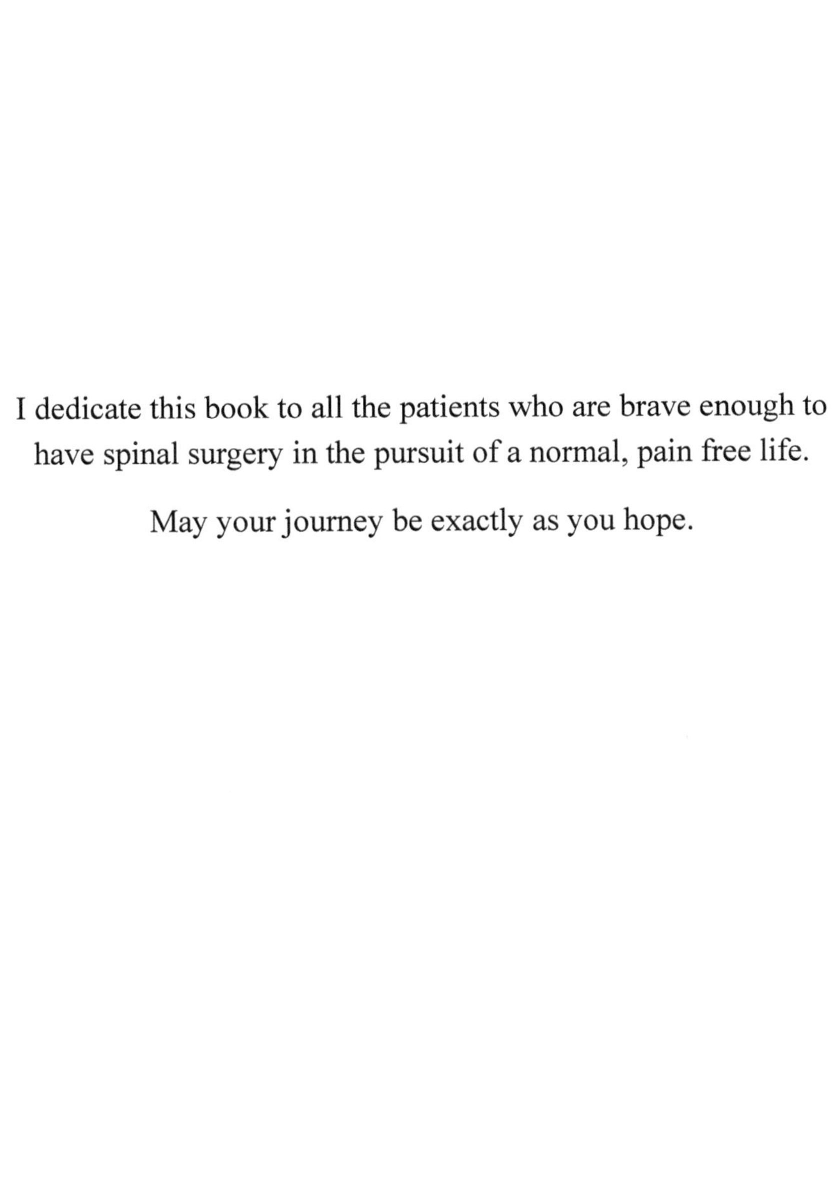

I dedicate this book to all the patients who are brave enough to have spinal surgery in the pursuit of a normal, pain free life.

May your journey be exactly as you hope.

Acknowledgements

I would like to acknowledge and thank profusely my surgeon, Dr Matthew Scott-Young, for his pioneering vision and his pursuit of excellence in all he does.

A massive thank you goes to the dedicated nurses and support staff at Allamanda Private Hospital on the Gold Coast.

Thank you to the many friends who plied me with well wishes, gifts, offers of help and visits. I appreciated every one of them and every one of you.

To Helen in our office – you made my absence possible by your dedication, professionalism and the capable way you handled everything. Your skills, friendship and trust are invaluable. Thank you.

Mum, your help with caring for the twins so that Darren could be with me for part of the time I was away was very much appreciated.

Thanks to our wonderful children, Robert, Michelle, Mark, Bradden, Samantha, Matthew and Michael for their constant love and concern throughout this process. I am truly blessed to have you all in my life.

An extra thank you to Sam for making time in your busy life to visit me every day in hospital; it meant a lot to me.

Another extra thank you to Michelle for coming to live with and care for me during my recovery – role reversal indeed! Your smiling face made my days.

My friend, Jo Munro, has my eternal thanks for flying to Queensland and spending five days upon my release from hospital nursing, cooking, caring, dispensing advice and, most importantly, making me laugh.

And finally, none of this would have been possible – not the operation, the recovery, the writing of the book – without the constant, unconditional and unwavering love, support and encouragement, both emotional and physical, of my best friend, my lover, my knight, my husband, Darren. To you I owe my life.

Claim Your Free Gift

To help you on your journey to becoming Pain Free, I've included a wonderful gift by International Hypnotist, Darren Stephens.

This amazing program, ***"Letting Go of Anxiety"*** (valued at $197) – one of 5 in the Pain Control Collection – is designed to help you overcome any anxiety you may be feeling relating to your back surgery.

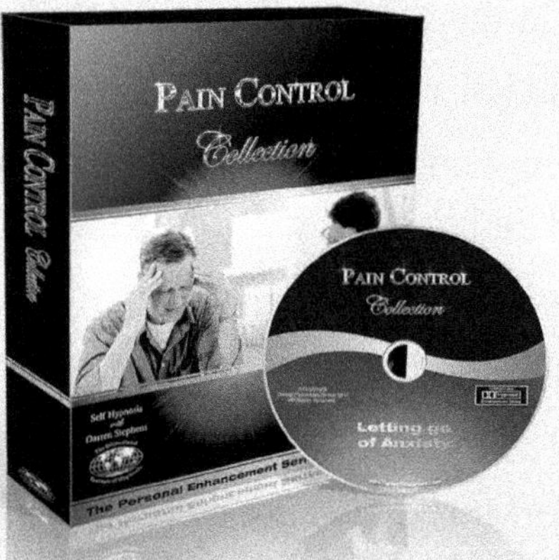

To claim your FREE downloadable CD, simply visit:
www.TipsForBackSurgery.com/Bonus

Contents

Introduction

So you're about to have, or you've just had, back surgery. Congratulations, soon you'll be very happy and doing things you haven't been able to do in quite some time. However, to get to that great place you've got to go through a time that is perhaps not as pleasant as you'd like, but totally necessary to get to the other side.

Remember, everybody's surgery is different. Some will have had posterior (through the back) surgery; some will have had anterior (through the front or tummy) surgery; some will have had disc replacements, some vertebrae fusions, some vertebrae drilled out and reshaped; the list goes on. I am not a medical practitioner; I don't know all the fancy names for the procedures and can't give you any specific advice about how to deal with your condition medically. Please, please, please ask your surgeon or physio (if you have one that is working in with your surgeon) for specific medical advice.

When I was getting ready for my surgery I was looking for "what do I need to do?" and "what can I expect?". I found that information in very short supply. Yes, there was information on the medical side about what was to be done and how my back would repair, but nothing on the practical side, like "how do I get my undies on if I can't bend to my feet?"

So, let's look at making your transition from back surgery to great health as easy as possible with some practical tips.

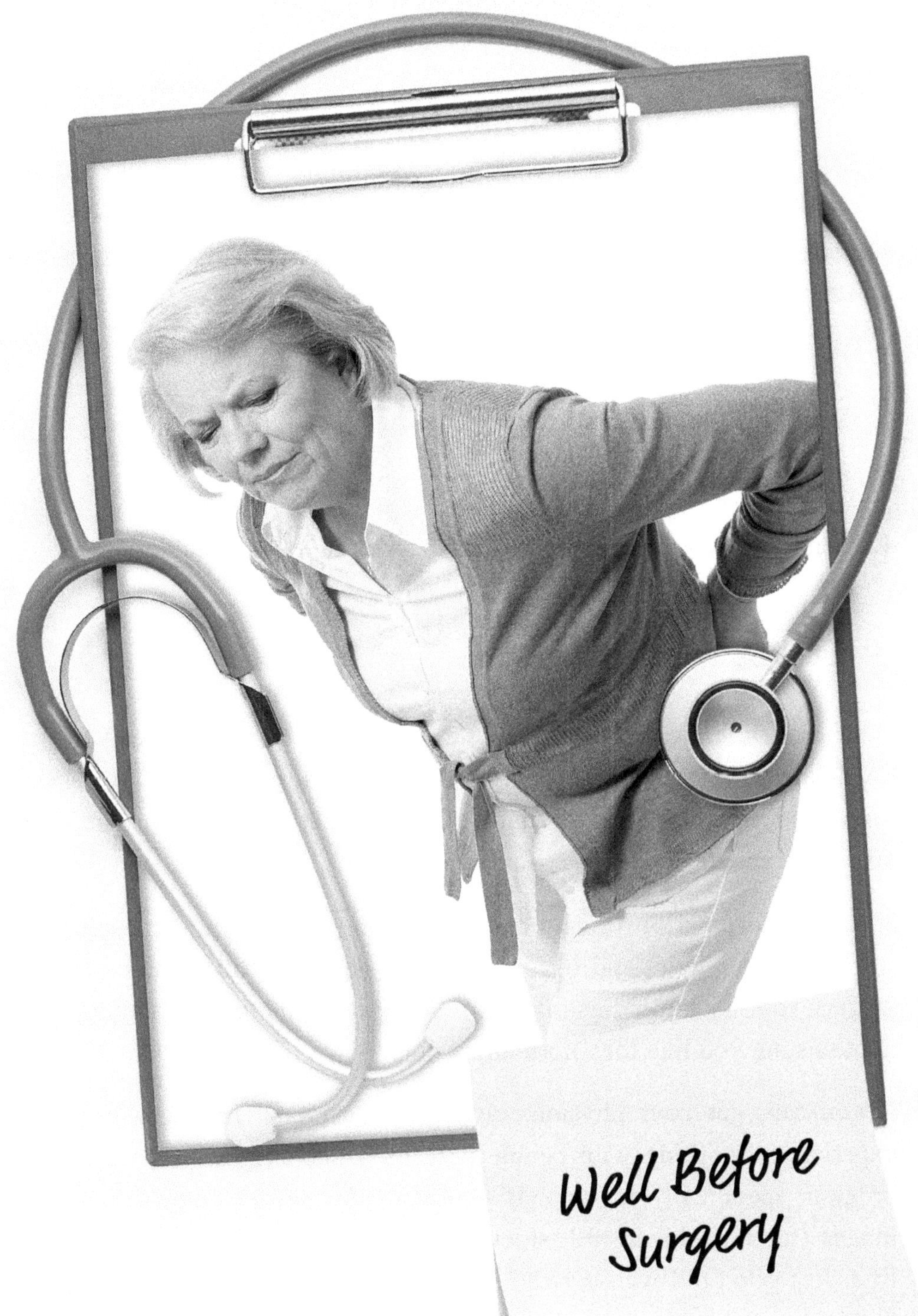
Well Before
Surgery

Well Before Surgery

If you're reading this and you've still got quite some time before surgery – fantastic! Here's four things you can do now that will help you enormously after your surgery.

1. Build up your leg strength
2. Work on your core and stomach muscles
3. Lose excess weight (if applicable)
4. Temporarily - or permanently - stop smoking (if applicable)

1 Build Up Your Leg Strength

When you first return home after surgery, extra leg strength will be invaluable to assist you in getting up from chairs, out of bed, off the toilet, and a myriad of other daily activities that you may currently take for granted.

If you've had anterior (through the front) surgery your tummy muscles won't be much help, and if you've had posterior (through the back) surgery your back muscles may be cut or a little traumatised and also not assisting you like they normally would.

If you can, get your physiotherapist, or a personal trainer who is experienced working with people with back challenges, to set up a program specifically for you. If you can't do that try some simple lunges (forward, backward, sideways), knee bends, toe rises or leg lifts. Just good old walking can also help with strength. Do nothing that hurts your existing condition. The idea is to strengthen your legs, not further injure your back.

2 Work On Your Core and Stomach Muscles

Having a strong core (the large group of muscles running through the centre of your body - primarily in your belly and mid to lower back) will assist you after surgery with everything from getting out of bed to quickly resuming your normal activities.

Again, a physio or trainer working with you is ideal. But if that's not an option, stomach clenches and isolations (either lying down or standing) and humps and hollows on all fours are a gentle start. Remember do nothing that aggravates your existing back issue. Walking also works on your core, as do most aqua classes; aqua aerobics, aqua pilates, deep water running. Aqua classes can be quite helpful as they generally allow exercise and resistance work without placing strain and pressure on already sensitive discs and muscles.

If your muscles are in good shape before the surgery it assists them to recover faster after the surgery, even if they've been cut.

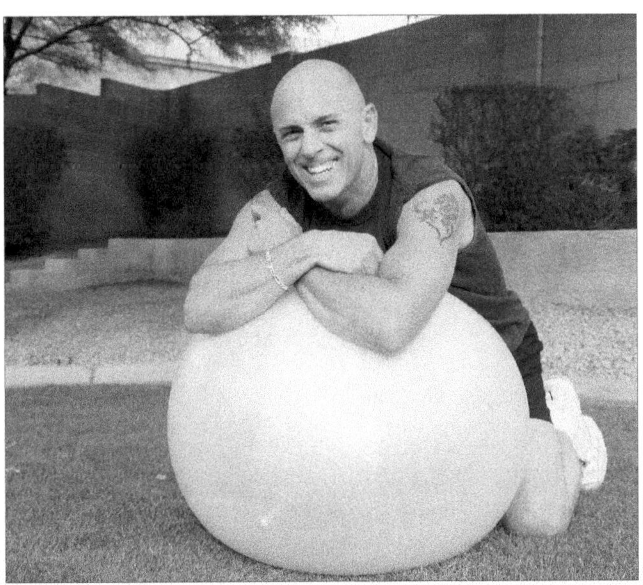

3 Lose Excess Weight (if applicable)

I don't know too many people who just love the process of losing weight; they love the outcome, just not the actions necessary to get there. However, if you're carrying extra weight, every kilo you can lose before surgery is one less kilo your back is going to have to support after surgery. It will be one less kilo dragging on your wound and stitches and one less kilo for your body to carry around when you want all your body's attention focused on healing and getting better. It's also better for you when you're under anaesthetic to be carrying less weight.

We know it's not easy; just do the best you can and remember that every little bit helps.

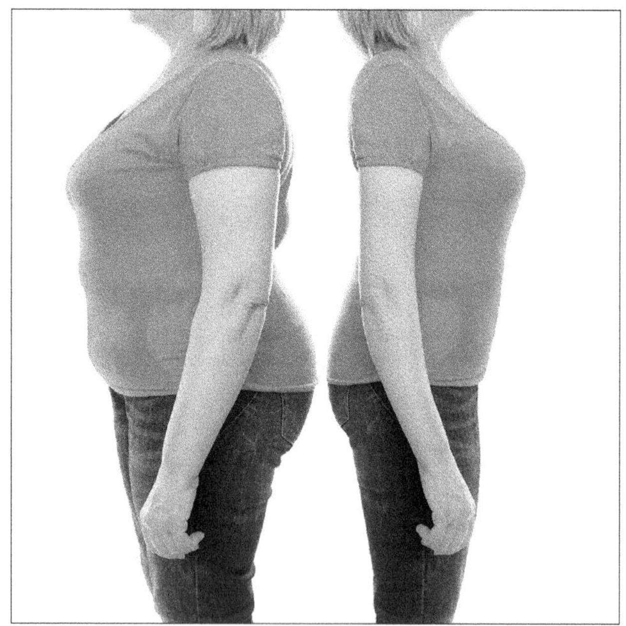

4 Temporarily - or Permanently - Stop Smoking (if applicable)

Again, this doesn't apply to everyone, and those it does apply to probably don't want to hear it, but stopping smoking as early as you can prior to your surgery will make a huge difference to how well you cope under anaesthetic. Those who smoke usually have lungs that are not working quite as well as they should (c'mon smokers, you know this is true). Under anaesthesia, it is better for you if your lungs are working more efficiently, as often lung function drops temporarily after anaesthesia (more about this in the next section).

It also aids in your healing process if your body is not diverting energy and resources to coping with smoke damage, but rather can focus fully on healing your back.

Like losing weight, it's not always easy, but there are many ways you can go about this: willpower, patches, hypnosis. Choose one that works for you.

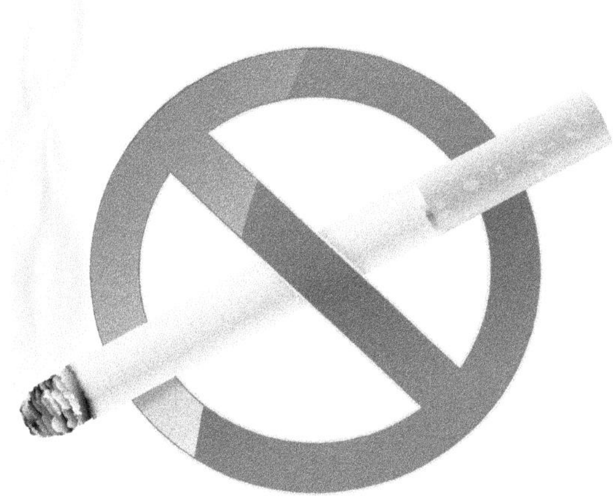

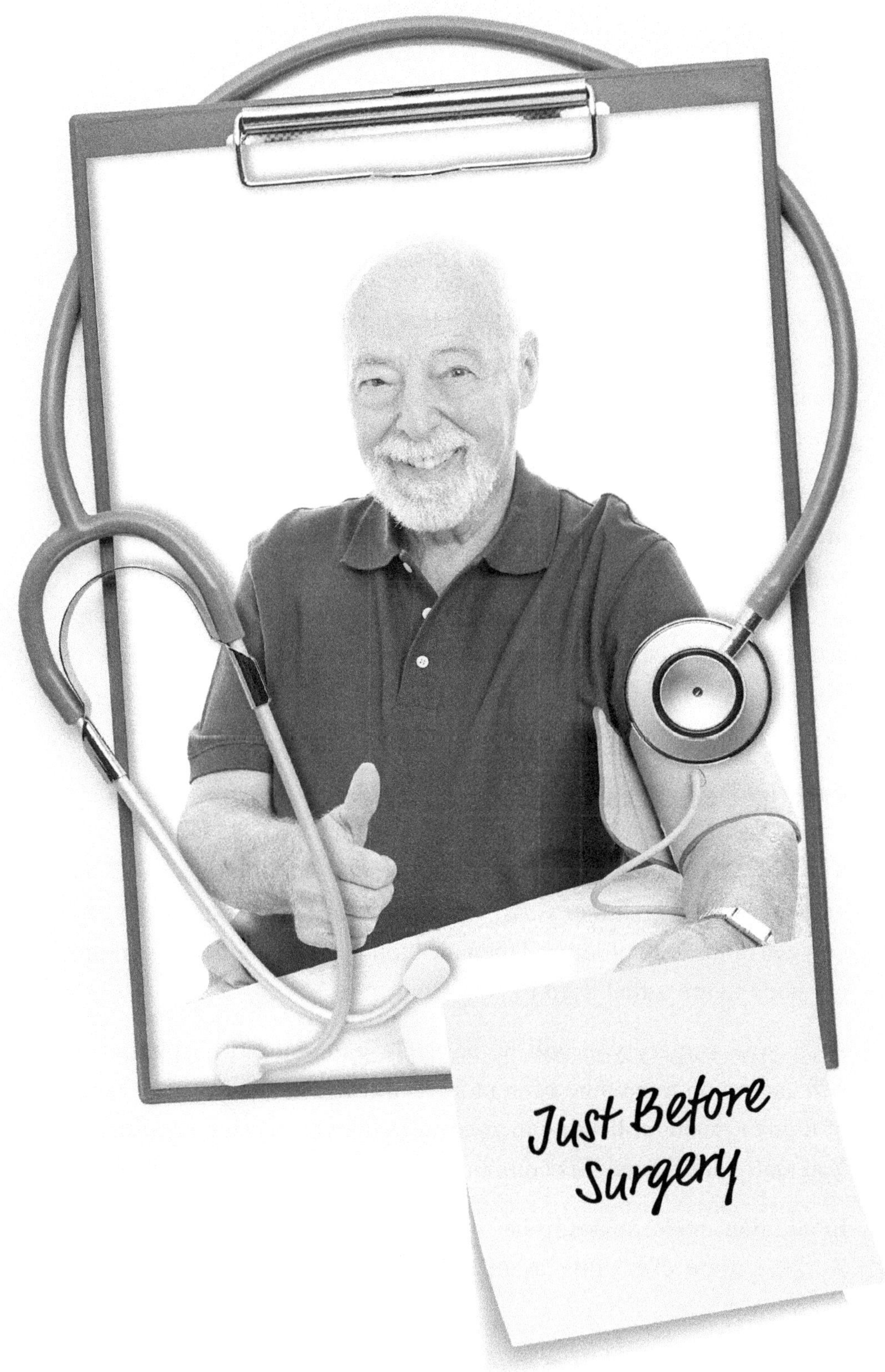
Just Before
Surgery

Just Before Surgery

Purchase all the items you'll need for when you're in hospital and all the items you'll need when you come out of hospital.

As you read further, you will find items I mention that you think will be useful for you. Add them to your "Shopping List" at the back of this book. If you are taking them in to hospital with you add them to the "Taking to Hospital List" as well.

Some things are easy to find locally and some you might choose to order online, so you need to allow delivery time. Remember that when you get home you will be doing lots of resting and healing. Shopping will be well down the list of things you need or want to do, and you probably won't be able to anyway. Be prepared and shop before you go in.

Practise Deep Breathing

Most of us shallow breathe into the top part of our lungs with the occasional deep breath or yawn when our body asks for more oxygen. Oxygen binds with blood and then the blood carries the oxygen around our body to areas that need it.

After your surgery you will be basically immobile in hospital. This will cause you to breathe even more shallowly, increasing the chance of fluid or mucus collecting in your lungs or even causing pneumonia. You really don't need this complication.

In addition, under anaesthesia, it is better for you if your lungs are working more efficiently as often lung function drops temporarily after anaesthesia.

Some hospitals will give you a little device with balls in it to help you practise and monitor your deep breathing (see right).

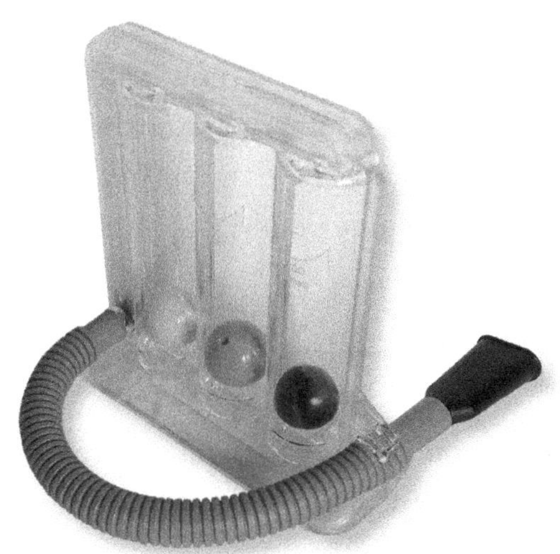

However, even without the device, you can do this on your own.

Simply cough all the air out of your lungs until there is none left, then take a very large breath in, feeling your lungs fill and your chest and stomach rise. Cough all the air out again and immediately take another deep large breath. Cough out, breath in. Do this for three or four breaths – no more or you may get light headed and dizzy. Do this every hour you're awake for a few days before entering hospital to get your lungs used to it. Then continue it in hospital while you're basically immobile.

Keep Yourself Healthy

Look after yourself before you enter hospital. Avoid burning the candle at both ends to get last minute things done for work or home. You want all your body's energy focussed on healing your back and the wound site, without it having to worry about just getting you back to a normal state after being sleep deprived or physically exhausted.

Likewise you don't want to come in with a cough or cold if you can help it. (Do you know how much it hurts to cough or sneeze when you've just had surgery?!) Look after your body, get enough sleep, take hot lemon drinks or vitamin C if that's something you do. Remember, you want to give yourself the best chance for a speedy recovery.

Fill Any Prescriptions You're Currently Taking

When you go in to hospital you will need to bring sufficient amounts of any prescription drugs you are currently taking to last your stay in hospital.

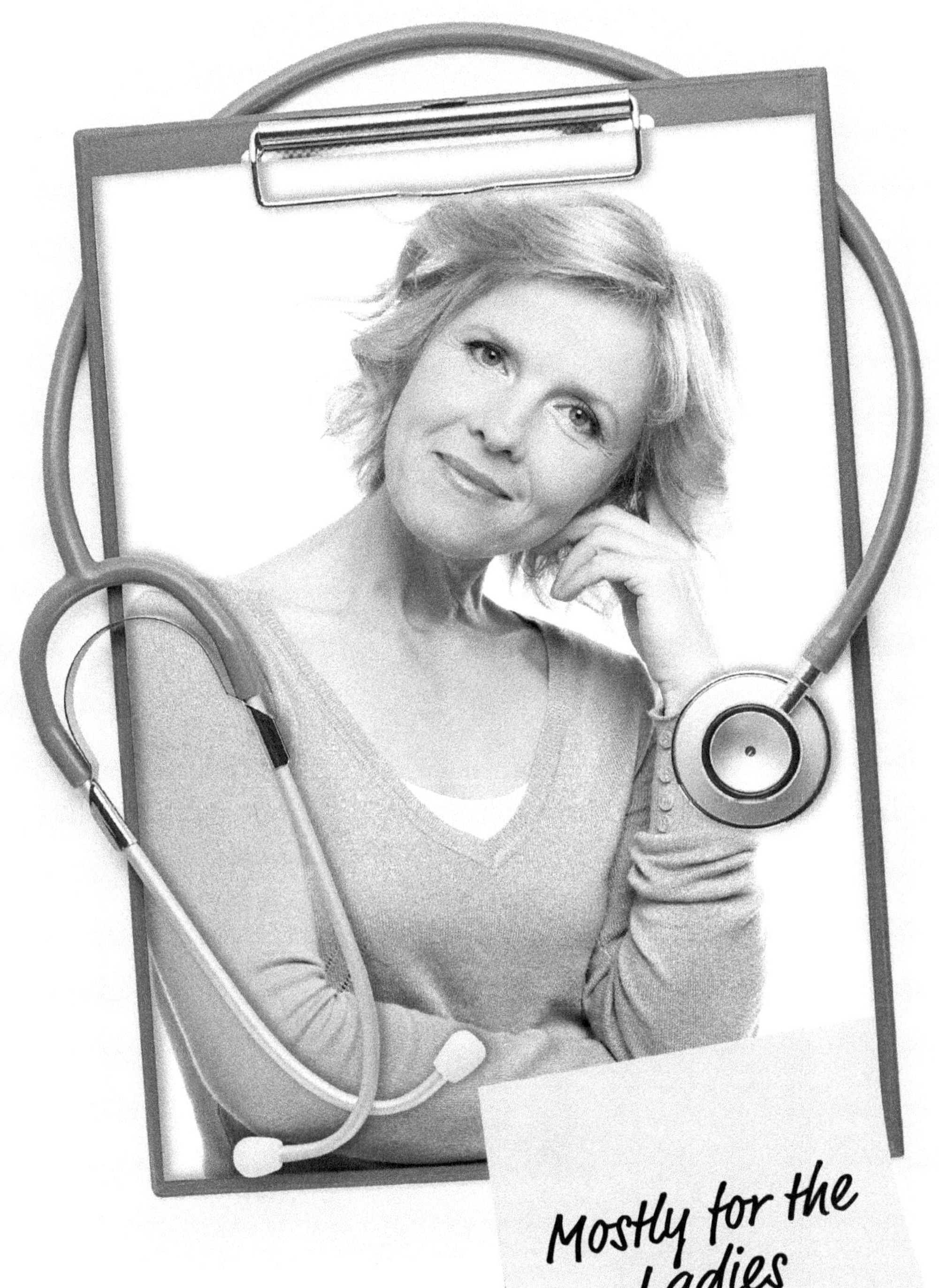
Mostly for the Ladies

Mostly for the Ladies

I'm going to be politically incorrect here and suggest this section is primarily for women, but if you're a gentleman who'd like to take this advice, please feel free.

Get Your Legs Waxed

You're not going to be able to reach them for a while, or be able to get up on, and down off, a salon bed, so get a wax and it will carry you through a few weeks.

Get Your Hair Coloured and Cut

When you come out of surgery you won't be feeling the best you ever have; you could be tired, nauseous and very sore. At least if your hair is neat, without a grey GT stripe down the middle, you won't also feel old!! It's also unlikely that you'll be able to sit in a hairdresser's chair for a few weeks so get it done right before going in to hospital to last you through recovery.

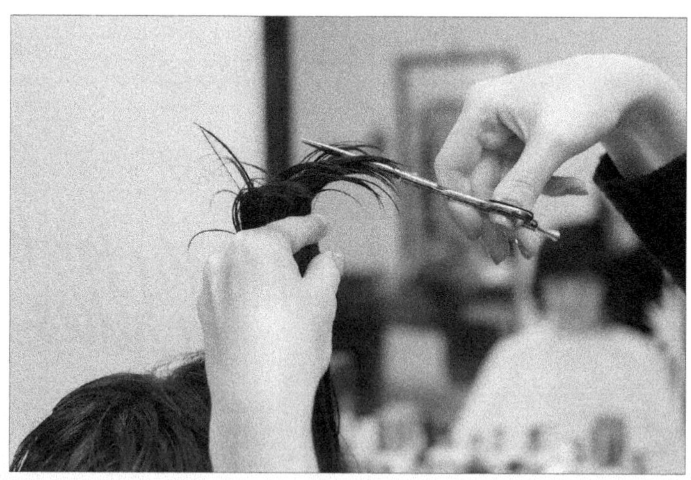

Remove Toenail Polish

a) Most hospitals prefer it to be off for surgery.

b) It will be quite a few weeks before you can get to your feet and by then it's likely to be looking chipped and ugly. Do yourself a favour and take it off now.

Waxing Other Areas

This one's a little more controversial and only applicable to some surgeries. If you're having anterior (tummy cut) surgery on your lower back, you're likely to wake up with the top half of your pubic hair shaved off. When it grows back it's prickly and sticks in to your tummy or legs when you're curled up. Some of you may prefer to wax the top half and avoid the prickle!

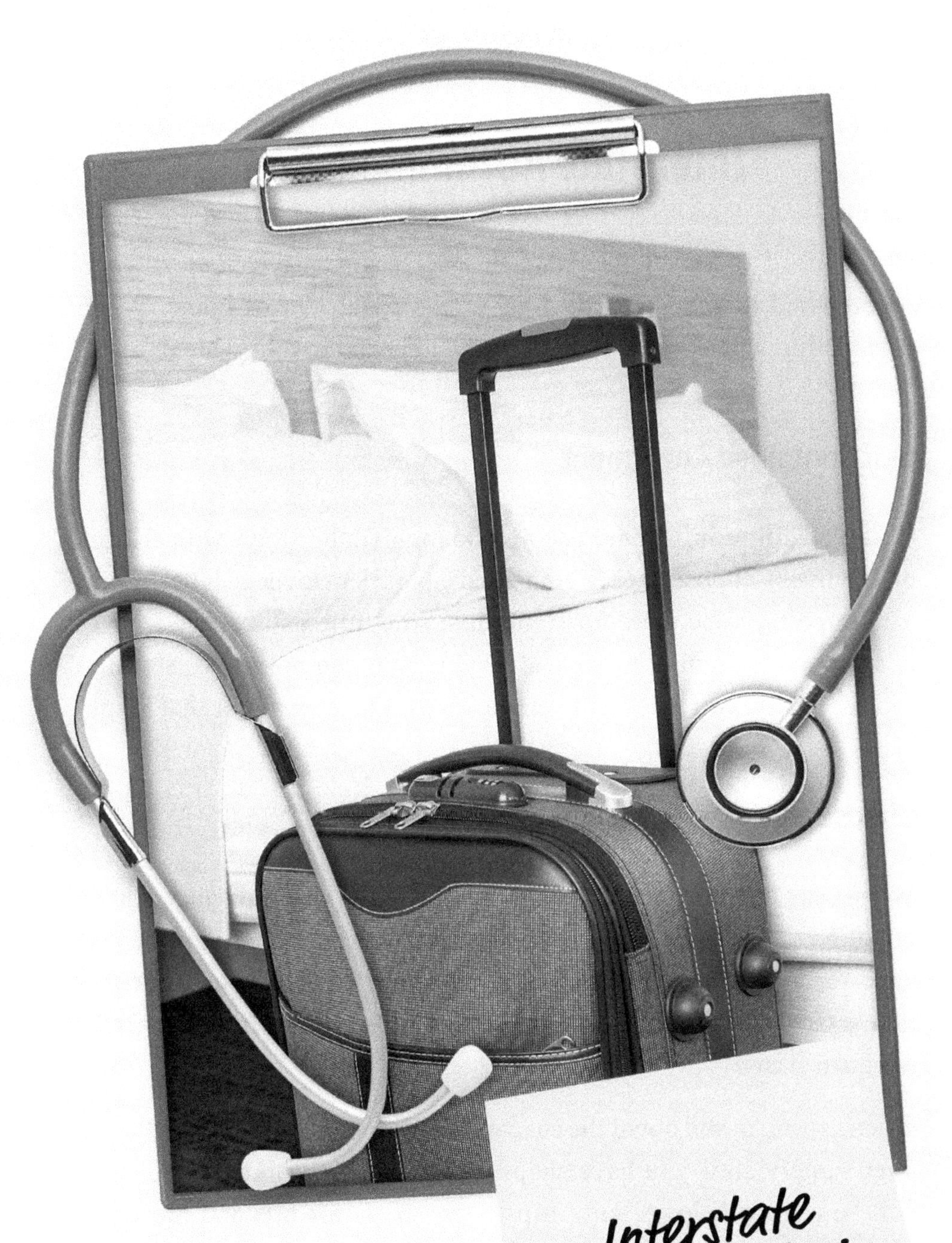

Interstate Accommodation

Interstate Accommodation

If you need to travel interstate or overseas to have your surgery, be prepared to spend two to four weeks living out of home. When considering where to stay you may like to keep the following in mind.

Self Contained Apartment

If you're going in to paid accommodation (rather than with friends or relatives) choose a self contained apartment over a hotel room. You're going to be there for some time so a little extra space is nice. If someone is coming to look after you, you can both have separate rooms. Lastly, you just don't want to live on take away for that long!

Choose a Central Location

When I say central I mean to the shops, not to the hospital. Once you're out of hospital you may not need to go back there at all, or maybe just once for a post op visit. You may only need to visit your surgeon's rooms once or twice, but you will need to get things from the shops on a regular basis.

Often getting in and out of the car can be quite challenging immediately after surgery so if you have shops within a short walking distance it will be a huge help. A daily trip to the shops for bits and pieces of groceries, or a meal out, will help you meet your walking quota as well. (See 'Managing and Keeping on Top of Your Pain', page 37).

Take a small, light back pack (if your wounds allow) as this is often easier than trying to carry plastic bags in your hands.

Elevators

If you're staying in any apartment style accommodation make sure there are elevators if you're on the second floor or above, or try to stay on the ground floor. In the early days your back may not like stairs very much.

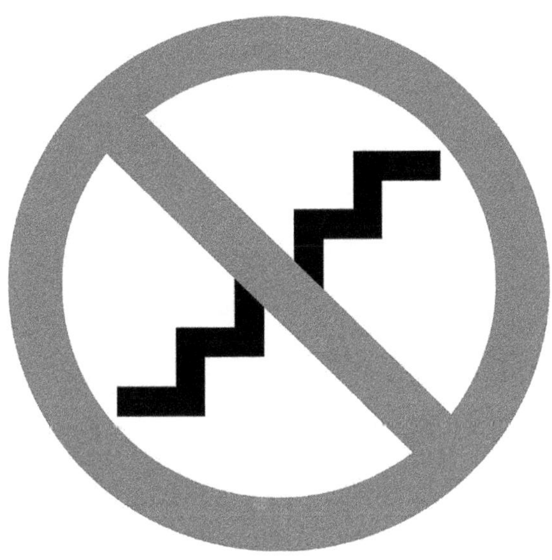

Walk In Shower

This one's essential if you've had lower back surgery. A lot of apartments have showers over the bath. Ask at the time of booking if they have any with walk in showers. Stepping over a bath will be difficult in the beginning. It also leads to a greater chance of falling (and you definitely don't want that!)

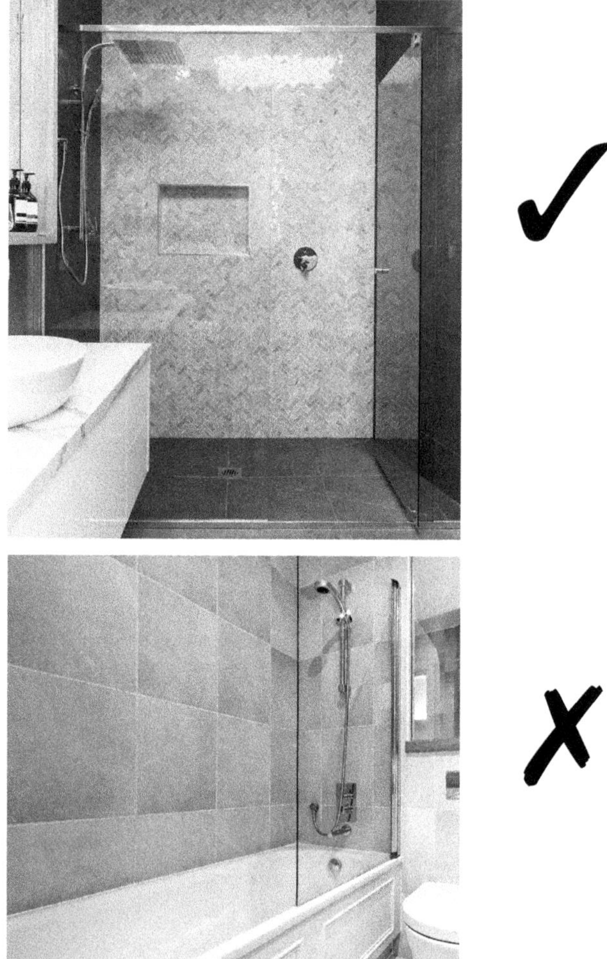

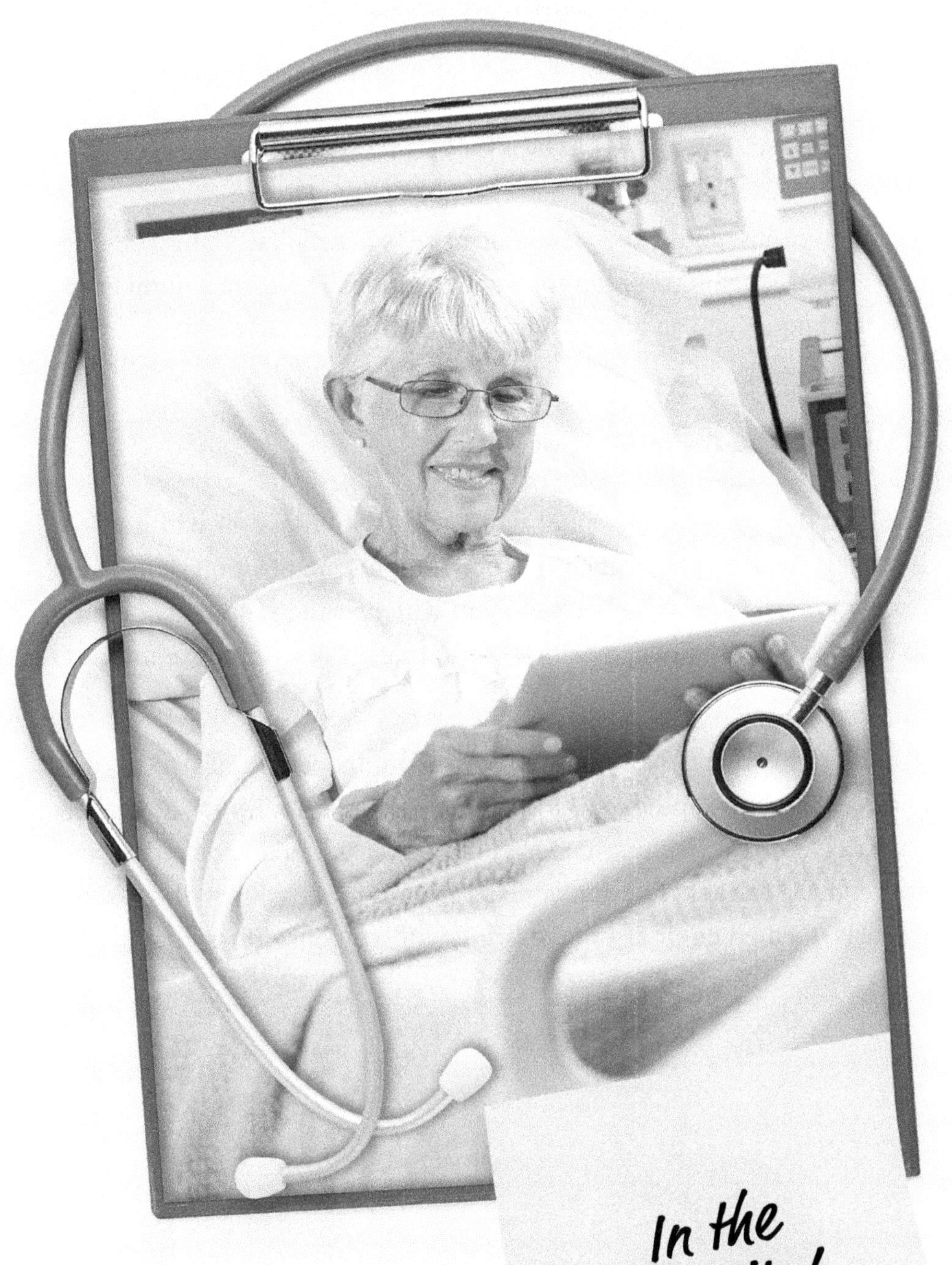
In the Hospital

In the Hospital

Some surgeries require only a couple of days in hospital, some a couple of weeks – ask your surgeon for a rough guide. There are a number of simple things that can make your time in hospital much easier.

Try Using a Body Pillow

The first day or two in hospital when you try to move, it will hurt so it's likely you'll spend much of your time in one position. However once you start to move in bed (and you will, because your body begins to hurt from being in one position) sometimes a body pillow can be of assistance.

A body pillow is one very long pillow about the length of two to two and a half normal pillows. It's useful for supporting your stomach, back, legs or just hugging under your head and can alleviate drag on your wound or back. Get someone to bring it in for you on day two or three as it's a bit cumbersome to bring with you on admission.

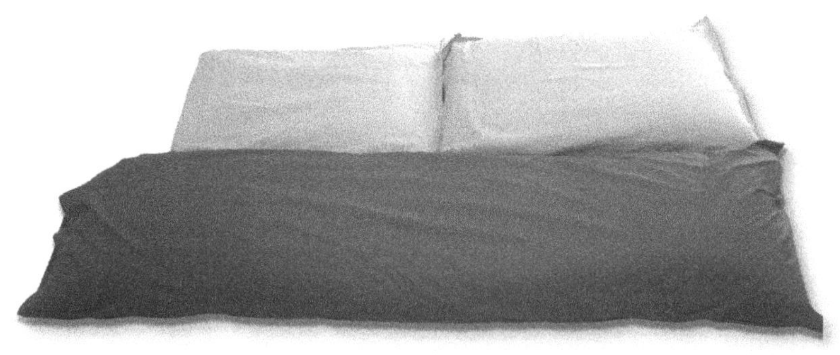

Use a Rolled up Towel for Relief

If a body pillow is too bulky for you or you just need a small lift, grab a clean towel and either roll or fold it in to the thickness you need. You can use it under your waist if on your side, or under the curve in your back if lying on your back.

Take Items for Entertainment

After the first day or two, when your anaesthetic and drugs have worn off, you'll be looking for something to do. Yes, there's always the TV, but there are only so many reruns of "Happy Days" and "Get Smart" you can watch. It can also be tricky to watch if the TV is mounted high and central and you need to lie on your side.

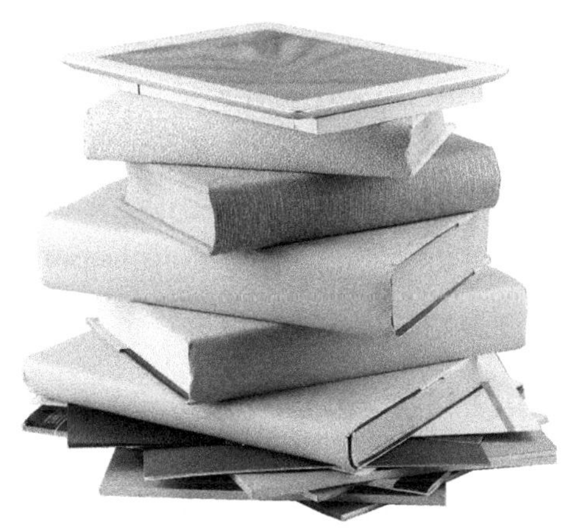

Get some books, magazines, puzzle books, Sudoku books or papers that interest you and take them with you so they're ready when you need them. You won't be walking to the shop to buy them and sometimes relatives, despite their best intentions, don't get what really interests you. Having something to occupy your mind also helps you to stop focussing on any pain you may be experiencing.

Some people take in paperwork to do (I was one of them) but I personally found this a little tricky. My mind wasn't quite on the ball and everything kept getting sprawled around and then moved as nurses came in to take observations, check my blood pressure, administer drugs, check wounds, etc.

A note on iPads – some hospitals don't like you bringing them in as they are a theft risk. Be aware of this and make your own decision bearing this in mind.

Take a Pen that Can Write Upside Down

As silly as this sounds, you'll be on your back or side a fair bit and normal pens stop working if held past horizontal. If you're doing puzzles or writing of any type do yourself a favour and get a couple of super thin Sharpie or Stabilo pens.

Shoes for Hospital

Take slip on slippers, sandals or thongs. You don't want anything with buckles, straps or heels. Most of the time you'll probably go bare foot anyway.

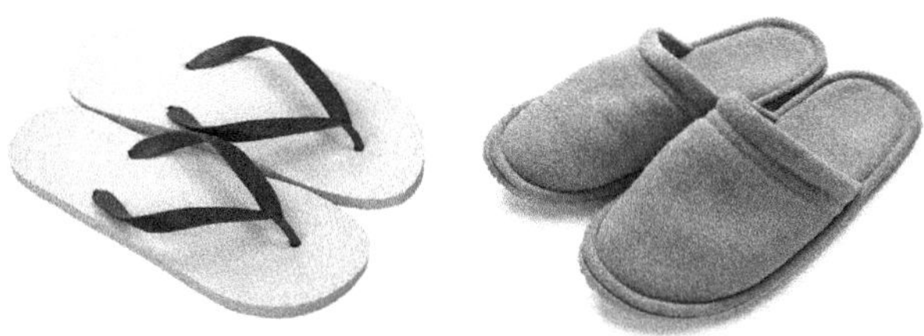

Soft and Loose Pyjamas

Now is not the time to be fashion conscious. Take in pyjamas or nighties that are soft and loose. “Grannie” nighties are ideal for women as they are roomy, gentle on your skin, usually cotton so you don’t overheat, and they won’t rub on wounds.

Loose Tshirt type tops and loose shorts are also good, remembering where your particular wound site will be. You don’t want tight elastic dragging across your wound.

On that note, because during the surgery your insides may have to be moved around and handled a little, you will possibly end up with swelling in that region. Allow for this and bring in larger than normal PJs. If you don’t own any, buy quite a few sets before your hospital stay. You want extras so that if your wound oozes or bleeds, you vomit, or spill things, you have fresh changes on hand.

Take a Slip on Cardigan / Windcheater

Hospitals are kept deliberately cool to assist in the prevention of germ reproduction. Sometimes you’ll get cold, especially once you start sitting up out of bed. Take something for your top half that is easy to get in to one arm at a time. Cardigans or zip up windcheaters are preferable to jumpers or sweaters.

Take a Set of Slightly Bigger "Going Home" Clothes

Parts of your body may still be swollen when you leave the hospital. Make sure the clothes you're going home in account for that. Try loose or elastic waist bands (or a loose dress for women). Now is not the time for your skin tight jeans.

Existing Medication

Take any existing prescription medication with you in their original boxes and place them in a large snap lock plastic bag with a short, written down list of what times you take them and give this to the nurses on admission. This keeps the medication and list all together but also stops any confusion as you will be groggy after surgery.

Take a Hand Fan

Sometimes your body will sweat a lot while you're in recovery. A hand fan is a quick and easy way for a cool down.

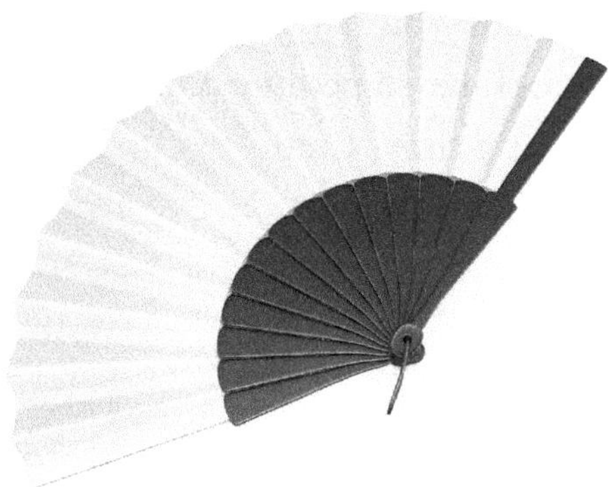

Take a Face Washer

Many hospitals no longer use cloth face washers; they use disposable cloths instead. Having your own real face washer is good for two reasons.

You can wet it with cold water and use it on your neck or face to cool you down when your body sweats.

If you normally use a face cloth on your face at home, the disposable ones are rough and don't do the same job.

Take Lip Balm (*Not* just for the ladies)

You will have had anaesthetic and an oxygen mask on, which will dry out your lips. You'll also be in full time airconditioning which is drying. Lip balm will help you avoid cracked lips and therefore eliminate one possible entry point for infection. Doctors and nurses will be the first to tell you that there are lots of germs in hospital. Do your best to guard against them.

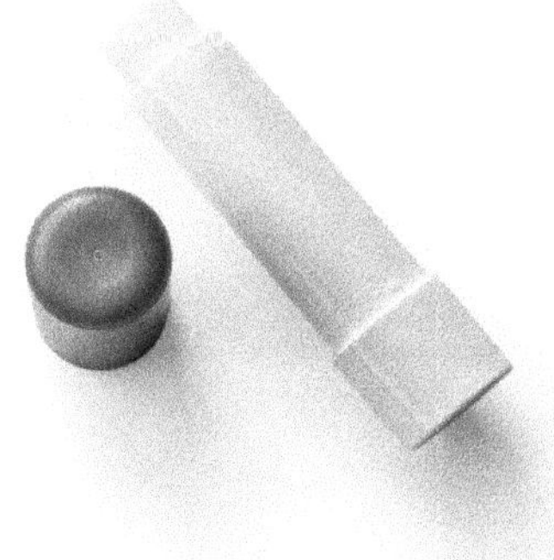

Protein Balls / Snacks

Even though they feed you in hospital, for a variety of reasons, the food is not always what you would like: it's different from your regular diet, or not as fresh, and/or not as frequent, etc. Take some healthy snacks with you or get someone to bring you in some fresh snacky fruit once you're allowed solid food.

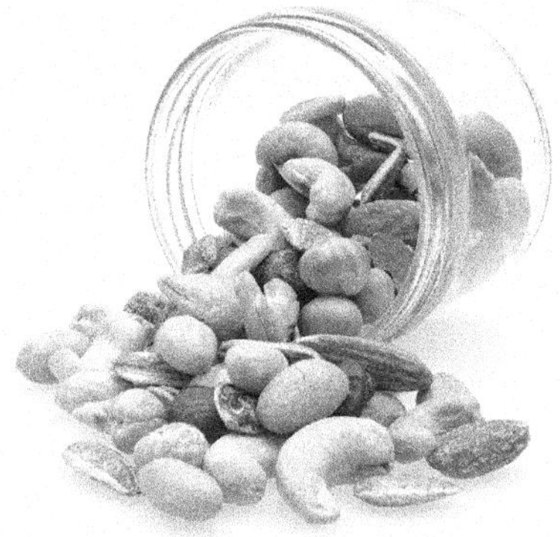

For those of you who like protein bars or balls, they are a great snack because, not only will they fill a gap but, they will also help you to heal faster. You need protein for muscle and tissue growth. Often the meals are not high in protein – especially if you are vegetarian. Another quick and easy snack is raw nuts: almonds, cashews, pecans, etc.

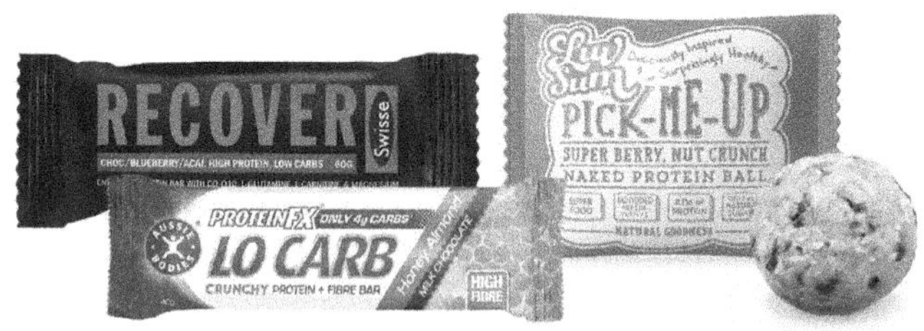

If you happen to be one of the unfortunate few who vomits after surgery, good old fashioned barley sugars are terrific. The little bit of glucose lifts you, is gentle, and helps take away the horrible taste in your mouth.

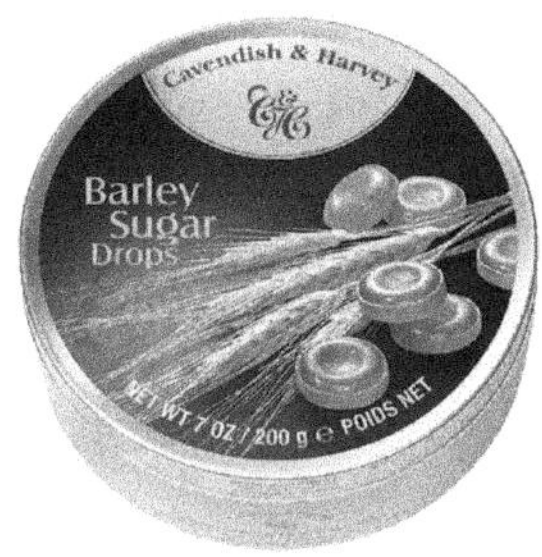

Have Roses in Your Room (Again *not* just for the ladies)

Not only do they look great and cheer you up, roses have an extremely high vibrational energy which some believe can assist with healing. Heck, if you don't agree with the healing side, they still look great, so what have you got to lose?!

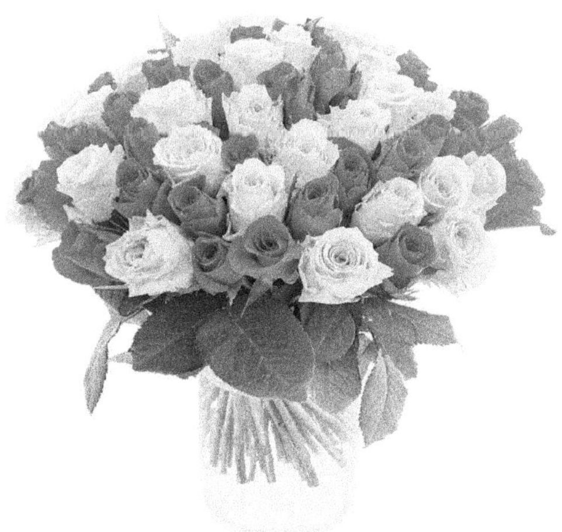

Have a Little Note Book Handy

Sometimes your brain can be a little foggy from the medications. Writing down your questions is a great way to remember them for when your surgeon comes in. Your surgeon is busy and their visits are likely to be brief and efficient so when they arrive, pull out your little note book and ask the things you might otherwise forget.

A second use for your notebook is to remember things that will need attending to in your real life outside the hospital.

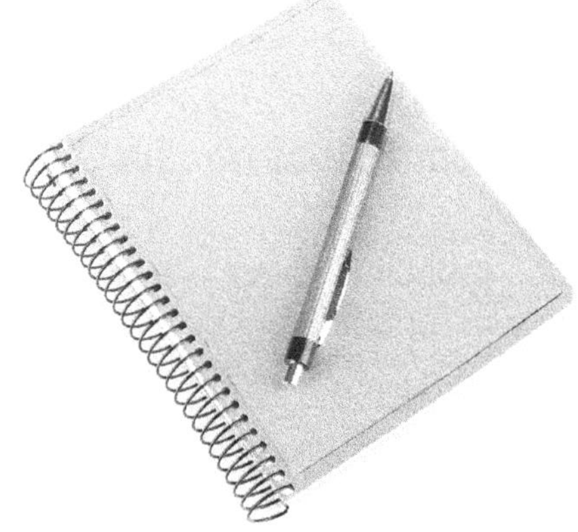

Sneezing / Coughing

If you need to sneeze or cough, bend your legs and support either your tummy or your back (depending on your type of surgery) before the sneeze or cough occurs.

The best way to support yourself is to grab a pillow and hold it in place firmly on your tummy or back, then cough or sneeze.

I know sometimes it's a bit tricky to get there in time, but trust me, after one painful cough or sneeze you'll be amazed at how quickly you can manage to get yourself in to a supportive position.

Sweating

Sometimes with very specific surgery using grafts to fuse vertebrae, you will experience an abnormal amount of hot flushes and sweating. This is actually a good sign that your body is healing. Even though there is nothing to fear, it can scare you a bit if you're not expecting it. If you fall in to this category, know it will happen and use a cool wet facecloth a lot on your face, neck, hands or other affected areas.

Physio / Rehab

It's likely that a physiotherapist or other rehabilitation specialist will see you after the surgery to give you exercises to help you get better (and stay better). Depending on the program in your hospital this may be a once only visit or daily visits. All I can say about this is **DO IT**. The success of your surgery and the amount of physio you do are directly related. Your surgeon has done his bit; now you need to do yours.

If you're told to do certain exercises four times a day, make sure you do them at least that many times. If they tell you to walk, then walk. If they tell you to rest, then rest. I know this sounds simple and like common sense, but many people ignore this part of their recovery and then wonder why they are not getting the results they would have liked from their surgery.

You've given up time and money to get to this point. Give yourself the best chance for success and do the activity the physio asks of you.

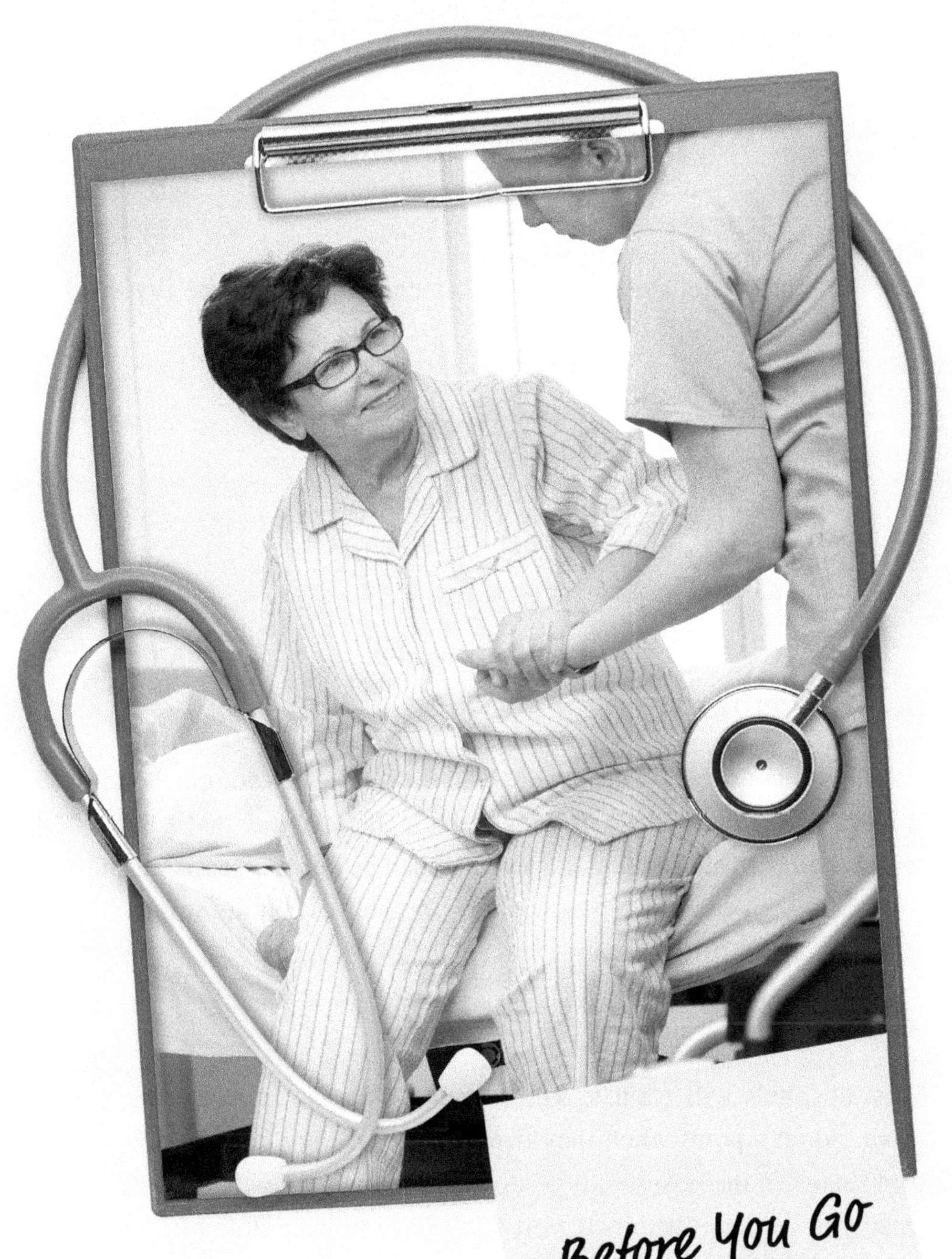

Before You Go Home

Before You Go Home

There is a myriad of medical things that need to occur before you leave hospital, but the four not so medical ones that you will be involved in are:

1. Walking by yourself
2. Walking up and down stairs
3. Passing wind (farting), and
4. Having a bowel movement (pooing).

1 Walking by Yourself

Usually on your second day in hospital they will get you up, even if it is just to stand by the side of your bed and, believe me, that's enough to start with. On subsequent days you'll then be taken on assisted short walks and then encouraged to walk by yourself within the ward.

2 Stairs

Most hospitals will want to know you can handle stairs before you leave. So, at a point when they deem you're ready you'll be taken to some stairs in the hospital to go up and down a few with supervision. Once you've done this once, you don't have to keep doing it; it's not training, just a little progress step you need to pass.

3 Passing Wind

Here's where I feel I should write two different tips. Most men don't seem to have a problem with farting; most women do. I have both male and female children raised in the same house with the same rules; the girls are reserved, private and polite about passing wind, while the boys think it is hilarious. My friends and colleagues report the same phenomenon.

However, in hospital you must pass wind and not try to stop it. It lets the staff know that air is now getting through your bowel and is the first step to bowel recovery (see the following point). You will be asked regularly if you have passed wind – answer truthfully.

4 Bowel Movements

You will not be allowed to leave hospital until you have had a bowel movement. This lets the nurses know that your bowel is back to operating normally. This is vitally important. During surgery, if your bowel is touched, it has a little spasm and may temporarily stop working. It usually starts up again all by itself and a bowel movement is the indicator this has happened. If it doesn't you could have a blockage or a twist in the bowel which may lead to nausea, giddiness and vomiting.

In addition to this, the anaesthesia and other drugs you have been given, or were already taking, may make you constipated. You don't want to have to strain with a fresh wound and a tender back, so either take in to hospital existing medication you are using for constipation or ask for something while you're there.

Remedies include teas (such as Bowel Klenz), tablets (such as Coloxyl or Sennesoft) or condensed chewable fruit products (such as Nulax). These are only some examples; there are many products. Ask your doctor or nurse for their recommendations. Also remember that you want something gentle on your bowel as explosive diarrhoea after surgery is not good either.

So, despite the fact that you may feel like a toddler going to a parent and saying “potty”, keeping track of, and informing the nurses honestly about, your bowel movements is critical.

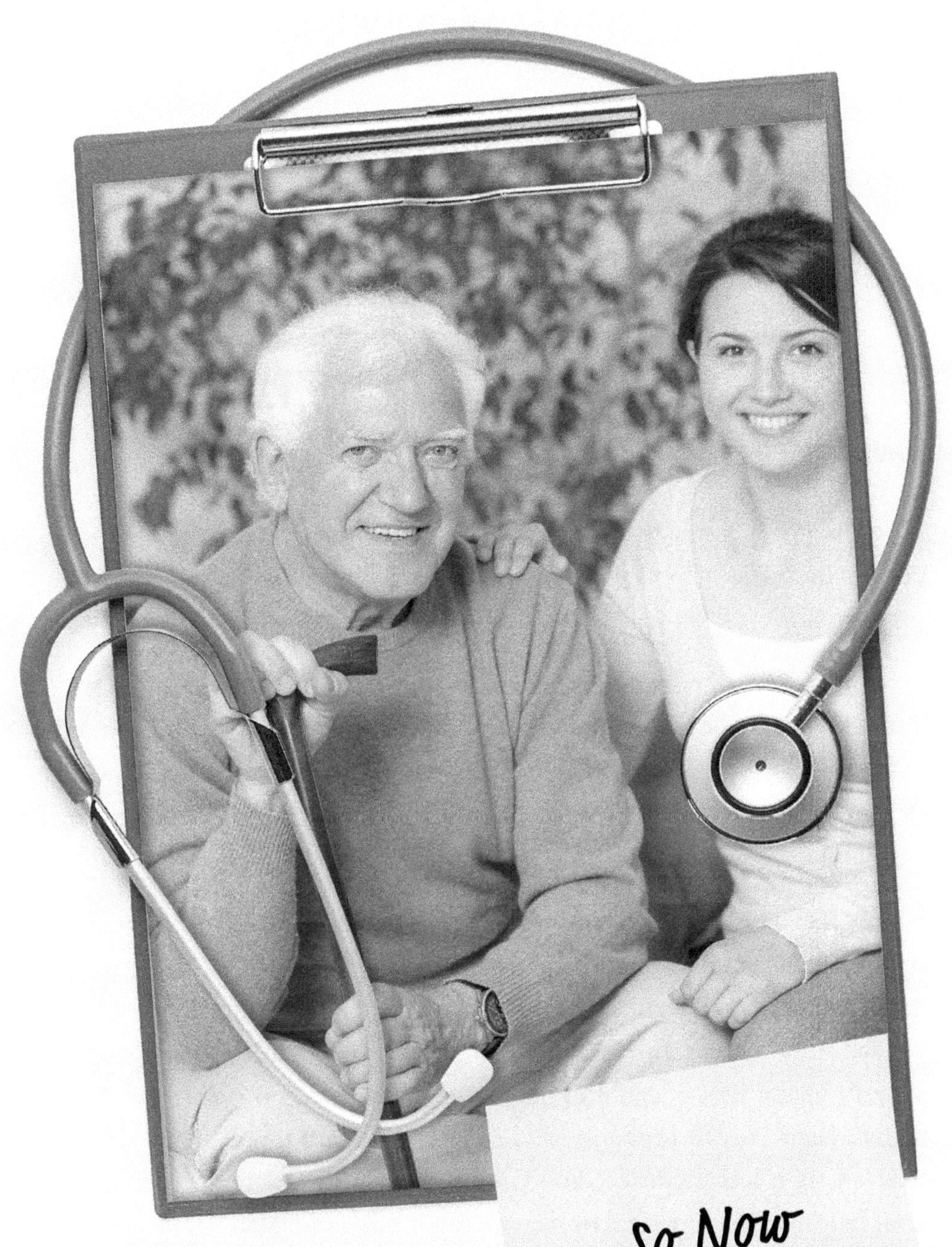

So Now You're Home

So Now You're Home

The catchcry you'll be given before you leave hospital is "No Bending, No Twisting, No Lifting" or a paraphrase of the same. With that in mind, let's see what we can do to make your life easier.

Have Someone Stay with You

If you're going home to a supportive and available partner, or a mature child – fantastic. If not, please ask a good friend, or a couple of them, for a favour.

When you first come home, at least for a couple of days, but preferably a week, have someone live with you to help you get settled and generally do things for you. The amount of assistance you need will depend on your type of surgery, but we all need a little help in the beginning.

I know it can be very hard to ask for help, especially if you're extremely independent and usually the person others come to. However, you have just had major surgery and you want to give yourself the best chance at a successful recovery, otherwise why did you have the surgery in the first place? Let people help you, even if only for a day or two each. You'll probably find your friends are more than willing to assist as it lets them feel good about themselves by contributing to you. Let them cook a meal or two, or fetch things for you when you're stuck in a chair and it's just too much effort to get up. Let them come with you for company, and support if needed, when you go on your rehabilitative walks. Allow yourself to be helped.

A Glasses Chain (if you wear glasses)

Let me say for the record, I hate glasses chains; they remind me of elderly aunts. I have to tell you though, mine became my best friend after the first time I dropped my glasses and couldn't bend down to pick them up. I couldn't read a thing until I got them back. Suppress any vanity you may have (or maybe that's just my issue) and wear one for a month or so until you are allowed and able to bend again.

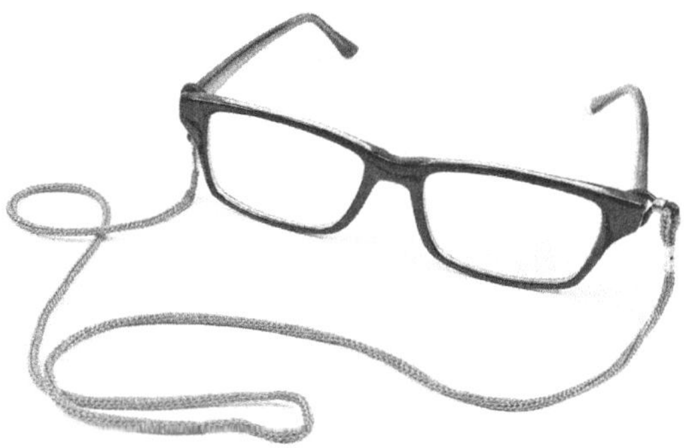

Two Soaps in The Shower

You're having a lovely shower when suddenly you drop the soap. You have two options – rinse only or call in your support person to pick it up. I didn't fancy either of those so opted for having two bars of soap in the shower. If I dropped one I simply finished my shower with the other. Once I was dried and dressed I could ask my friend to pick up the dropped soap so I had two ready for next time. Another person I know went for the soap-on-a-rope option.

A Long Handled Body Brush or Body Sponge

If you want to wash your feet or lower legs unassisted, then buy a long handled body brush or body sponge and put it in the shower. Soap the sponge or brush and slowly lift one leg slightly and sponge down that leg, then do the other. The first few days, even this may be too tricky and so a rinse might be all they get.

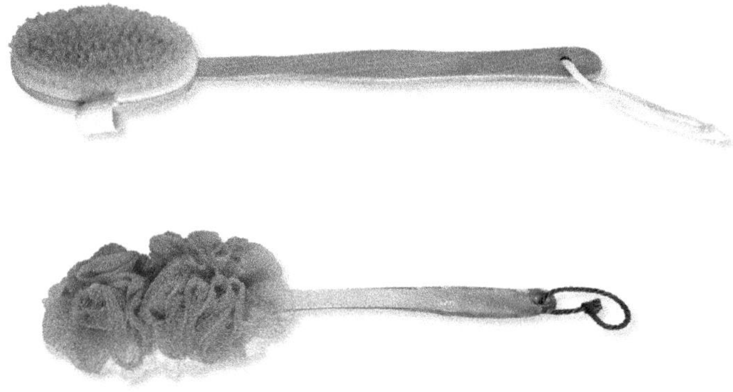

A Plastic Stool in the Shower

Let's stick with the shower theme for a moment. A simple plastic stool of knee height or above that you can pop in the corner of the shower is a wise investment. When you first come home you are likely to be a little weak and sometimes the extra heat and steam from the shower can make you feel a little light headed. I always found plonking myself on a stool for a few minutes preferable to having my care person come in and have to pick me up naked and wet off the bathroom floor.

Some people have also used the plastic garden chairs. I personally found these a bit bulky and a little awkward if you actually need to wash yourself, but they're still a good second choice.

Drying Yourself

You've survived the shower – now for the drying. The top half to groin level is easy but suddenly your legs and feet are out of range. Here's some tips for managing without hurting yourself.

To dry the tops of your legs to knee level carefully lift one foot on to the toilet seat. This allows you to rub the top of your raised leg on both the front and back. Swap legs. For the bottom half of your legs, again put one foot carefully up on the toilet lid. Holding one end of the towel in one hand and the other end of the towel in your other hand, hook it down past your knee like a sling and slide the towel from side to side – shin dry! The same can be done for the back of your leg – calf dry. And swap legs.

Put a towel, or towelling bath mat, on the floor that you can leave there. Wipe your feet on it thoroughly like a door mat, then scrunch up a little section of it in to a small lump with your toes. This allows you to dry behind your toes.

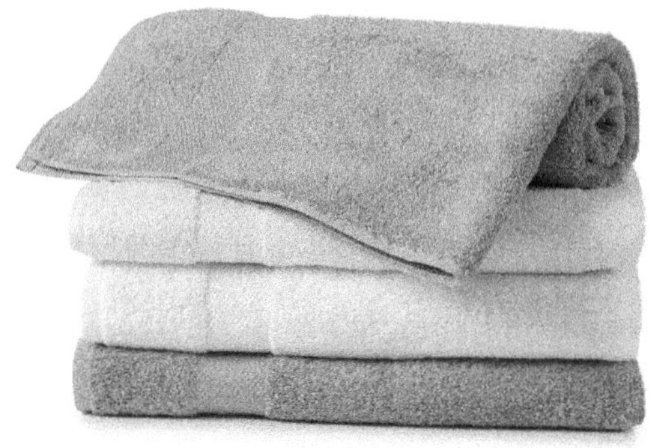

Getting Your Undies On

This topic raised much discussion and sharing of ideas amongst those I was collaborating with. There was discussion about how true your friends were if they helped you get your undies on, whether you even could or should ask them, and the general consensus that most friends would be fine with helping. No matter how we looked at it, we all agreed we'd rather do it ourselves.

The following was seen as the easiest, least painful method, and gave the most consistent results (ie. getting your undies on).

Sit on the toilet (or side of the bed if it's low enough). Hold on to the waistband of your underpants on one side with the opposite leg hole dangling down between your legs. If your seat is low enough you should now be able to swing your undies and hook your toes, and then your whole foot, in through the leg hole. Pull them up almost to knee height. Then, hold the waistband at the side you've already got on and then lift and hook your second leg in. Pull to above knee height. Stand up, pulling the last bit up as you stand and there you go – undies up and dignity intact.

Loose and Low Undies

While we're on the subject, if you've had lower back surgery, buy yourself some cheap cotton undies that you know you'll only wear for the next few weeks. Get them a size or two bigger so they won't rub, and get a "bikini" style (men too). These will sit low on your hips and under your tummy. This prevents rubbing across your hospital dressing, and your wound when the dressing comes off.

Toilet Lids and Seats

No matter what the rules have been previously in your home, for a few weeks you need to be able to leave the toilet lid up. Most toilet lids when closed are too low for you to lift up without bending.

The same applies to the toilet seat. If you're a female who's had surgery you'll want the seat down, and a male who's had surgery will mostly want the seat up. Make sure all members of your household, including kids if you have them at home, are made aware of your need to have the seat a certain way. If people forget you can always, at a pinch, lift the seat with your knee.

Have a Cup in the Bathroom

If you're a person who scoops up water in your hand to rinse your mouth after toothbrushing, it's unlikely you'll be able to bend over to get the scoop to your mouth without it dribbling all over you. Put a cup beside the sink. Also, when spitting after rinsing, it will splash back up on your tummy. Spit in to the cup, then tip it out and rinse the cup out. Soon you'll be able to squat down enough to scoop and spit.

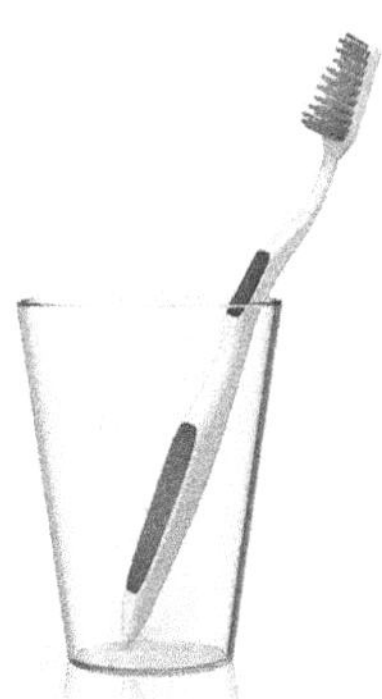

Using a Four Pronged Cane

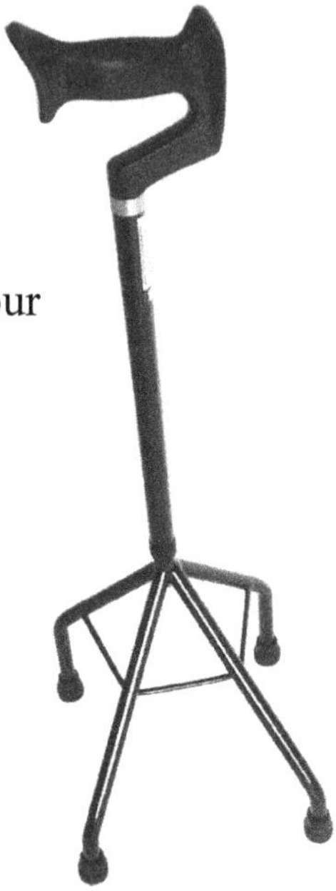

You won't need, and shouldn't use unless instructed by your doctor, a cane for walking. What it IS fantastic for is helping you get up out of a low bed or low sofas and chairs. Put it squarely on the floor in front of you, between your legs, and lean on it for leverage to get up.

You can carry it from room to room if needed and the four prongs give it a nice stable base without taking up a lot of room.

These can be found online, at large chemists or medical aid shops.

Long Handled Pick ups or Pinchers

I've included photos of two samples – one inexpensive and one more solid so you know what I'm talking about.

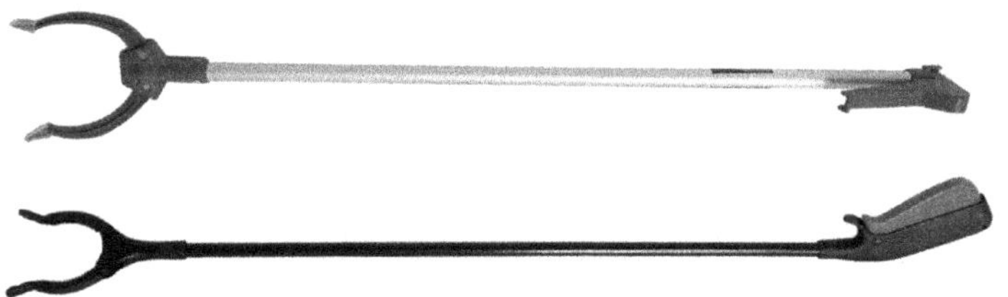

This little tool was an absolute life saver when no-one else was in the house. If you drop things like tissues, clothes, food, anything at all, it allows you to pick them up again without breaking the "no bending" rule. Again, online or medical aid shops and chemists are your best sources.

Move Things Up in the Fridge

While the pinchers can be used to get low lying things in your fridge, the items can sometimes be a little heavy. Either before you go in to hospital, or with the help of someone when you come home, move the items you use to the higher shelves or the door.

Prepare Small Meals

Because your stomach may have been upset in hospital and because of the natural tendency of your bowel to be moving slowly after surgery, smaller amounts of food more often will be easier on your digestive system. You can have smaller snacky types of meals or cook standard size meals and split them up so they can be eaten over time rather than all at once.

Have Fruit on Hand

Because fruit is easily digestible and can be readily eaten in smaller portions, it is a great option. If you're not in to apples and oranges, try passionfruit, kiwi fruit, grapes, cherries, raspberries, mangoes or strawberries.

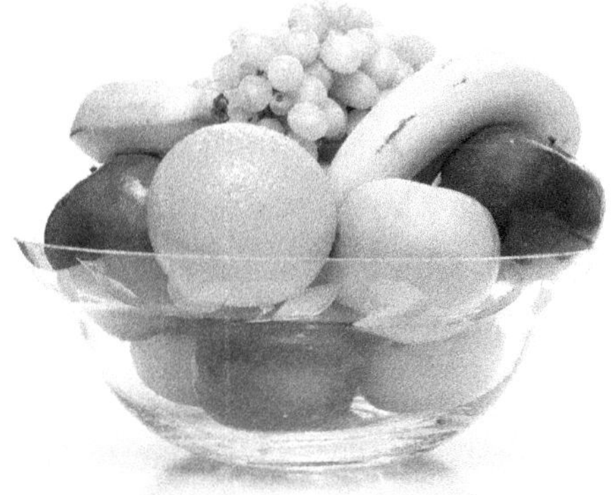

Have Juices on Hand

Again, juices are an easy way to get much needed nutrients in to your body in a more gentle way. If you have a good vitamiser or juicer you can make your own. If you don't want to make your own there are plenty of commercial juice bars. Also many freshly squeezed and combined juices are now available in the supermarket.

This is especially good if you're one of the few whose bowel is taking longer to get back to normal.

Have Sick Bags on Hand

If you vomit in hospital they will have sick bags on hand. This is not as uncommon as people think; your body has been traumatised and it is also trying to get rid of the anaesthetic and other drugs.

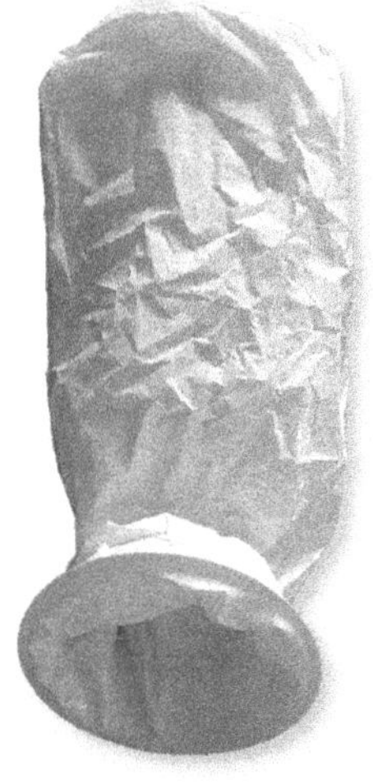

The same bags you use in hospital can be purchased online or from chemists quite inexpensively. One example is "Chuckies". These are a plastic bag with a solid plastic round lip. Once you have been sick in it you simply twist it closed, sealing in the mess and smell, and then dispose of the whole bag. There is no rinsing out containers or having to mop up spills. This is far better if you're by yourself, as well as for the person caring for you.

Some of you will not vomit at all but some may for a variety of reasons: reaction to medication, bowel not working properly yet, your body getting too hot, amongst others. For my way of thinking it's better to be safe than sorry (and it turned out I needed them!)

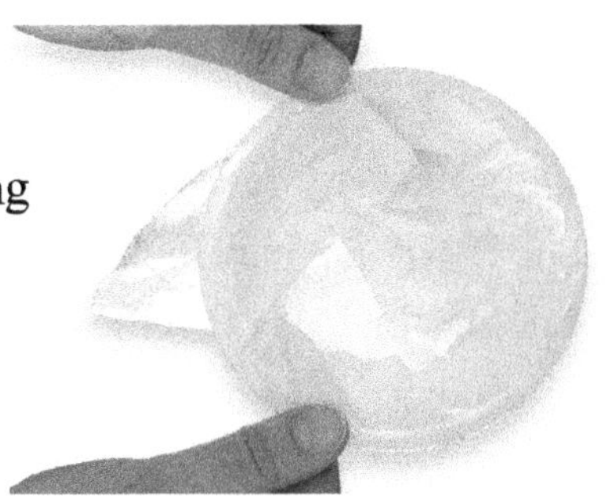

Have a "Sippy Cup" or Bendy Straws

While you're spending time in bed, not having to struggle to sit up every time you want a drink of water is a blessing. Packets of bendy straws are in most supermarkets and often straw cups or sippy cups (ones with a spout) are as well. Let your inner child out for a little while!

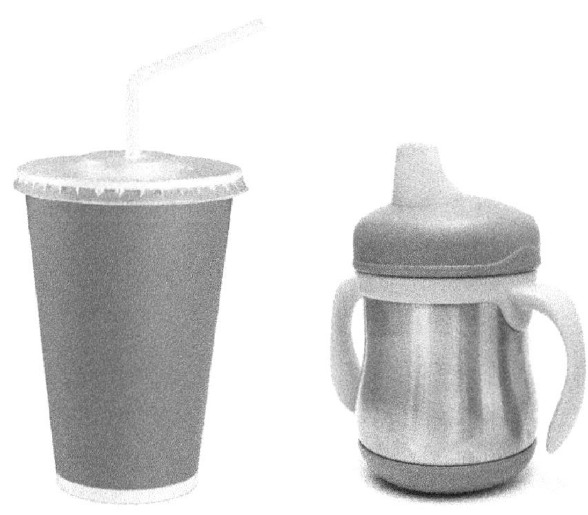

Slip On Shoes

Do yourself a favour and wear thongs, slip on sandals, slip on casual shoes, or go barefoot if you can. It's unlikely that you'll be doing buckles or laces for a few weeks unless you plan to ask someone else to do them for you. Ladies, please stay away from the heels.

Pressure Stockings

It's likely you'll be made to wear pressure stockings (long socks actually) while you're in hospital. You should ideally wear them for the first couple of weeks at home as well. Because you're more immobile than usual, your chances of getting DVT (deep vein thrombosis) are increased. This is a simple, if not particularly glamorous, way of helping to prevent that.

Most nurses will say to wear them at night and take them off during the day if you're being reasonably mobile and walking. You will need help to get these on and off as, if they're fitted correctly, they are extremely tight.

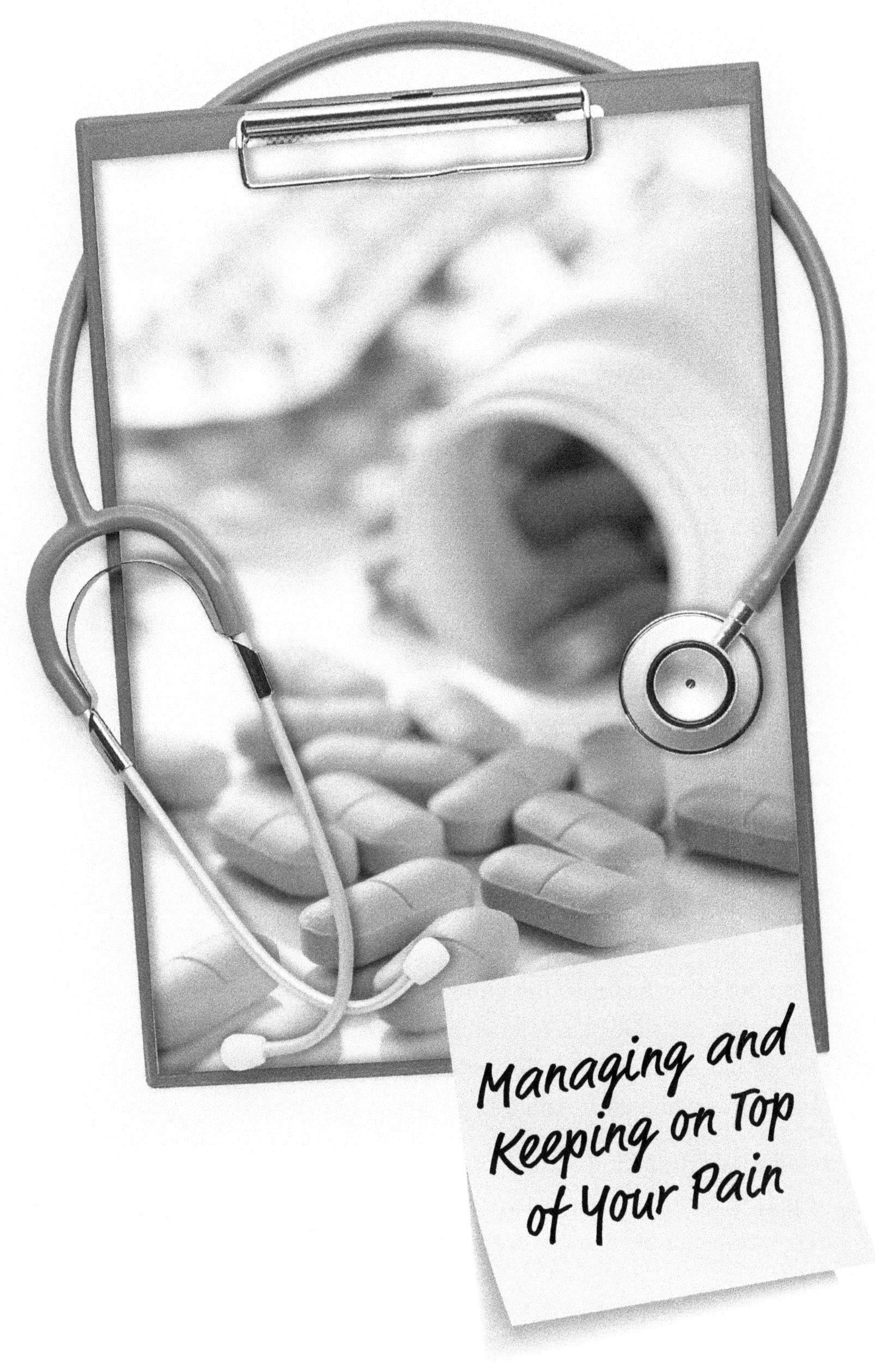
Managing and
Keeping on Top
of Your Pain

Managing and Keeping on Top of Your Pain

Stay on Top of It

I've always been, for better or worse, a "suck it up" type of person. The standard response in our house to any type of illness complaint has always been "Have a big glass of water, go to bed, sleep, and you'll feel better in the morning". Nine and a half times out of ten it works; sleep is a great healer – unfortunately not after major back surgery.

I took the time to become quite educated around current medical thinking on pain management. Here is my very simple, non medical and paraphrased explanation as I understand it. Think of your pain as a line on a graph climbing higher and higher if left unattended. Eventually it passes an invisible horizontal line which is your particular level of pain tolerance. What happens now is that you are in what you consider to be extremely high and often unbearable pain. To get you back down below that line takes lots and lots of pain medication, and maybe different varieties, and a bit of trial and error to get the mix right.

If, on the other hand, as the climbing pain line is going up, but still under your invisible pain tolerance line, you take medication to assist, you would need a much lower dose to keep your pain line from climbing any higher; it would level out or perhaps drop a little.

In other words, taking a small amount of medication at the beginning of pain symptoms is far better than having to take lots of medication to try and get it back under control if you wait until you're in agony.

This went against my own personal philosophy of "toughing it out" so, of course, I tried the hard way first until I realised I was having to take more drugs rather than less.

In short, it is better to take lower dose medication at the onset of pain to stop it getting away from you.

Take a Rapid Release with a Slow Release

If you're taking something simple like Panadol for break out pain between your prescription meds, consider taking one rapid release and one slow release (like Panadol Osteo). This gives you a quick acting relief with a long term relief at the same time and can help you manage a little better. When this was suggested to me it definitely made a difference. Discuss it with your doctor or pharmacist.

Set a Phone Alarm for Your Meds

Prescription medication for back surgery is often slow release. For example, the medication may be a 12mg dose which you take twice a day. This means that your body is getting about 1mg of that drug every hour. It's designed to stop your pain from getting away from you (as discussed previously). If you don't take the medication at the time you're supposed to (after all, what difference does a few

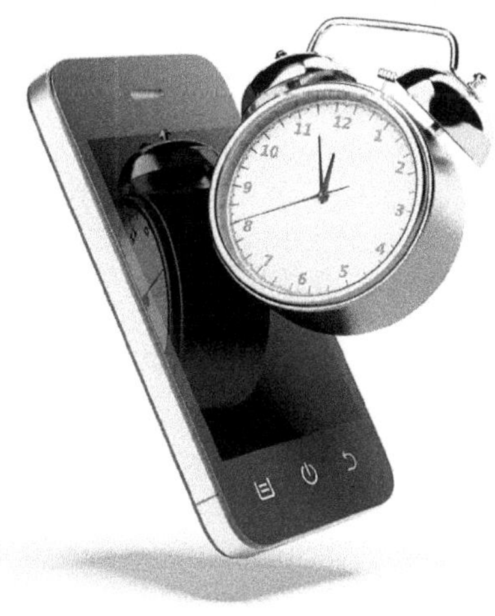

hours make??) then you're actually messing up the nice even pattern of slow release and causing your pain line to climb up and drop back. Remember, what you want is a nice smooth horizontal or slightly decreasing line.

I'm not good at remembering to take tablets (mostly because I subconsciously don't want to) and so found the easiest way to remember, and therefore get the best results, was to simply set a recurring alarm on my phone for the time, morning and night, when I needed to take them.

Heatbags / Icepacks

Aches in your back and legs can be extremely annoying and sometimes stop you in your tracks. A microwavable heatbag, a good old hot water bottle in a cover, or an icepack in a towel are all wonderful for easing those aches. The medical professionals I spoke to said there were mixed feelings about heat v cold so to do what felt best for you.

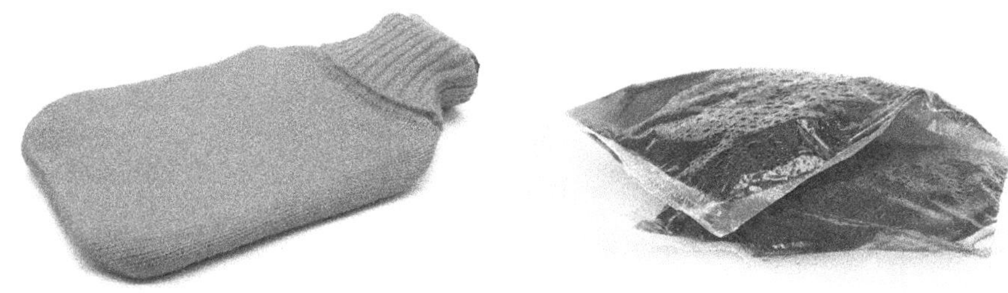

Walking / Sitting / Lying Down

After back surgery if you lie down too long you hurt, if you stand up too long you hurt, if you sit down too long you hurt, and if you walk too much you hurt. Here's the interesting and ironic thing – you need to do all of them and rotate through.

You must stand so your back can get used to your new structure and posture. You must lie down so you can rest and heal. You must walk to encourage all the muscles and internal structures to repair. You must sit so your body becomes acclimatised to this position.

In other words, you need to do them all, but in moderation and changing position often.

Back Support Cushions

There are a large variety of these on the market, from the inexpensive discount store variety to the highly engineered higher end variety (such as Comfyback) available from your physiotherapist, or online. These assist with your posture whenever you're sitting and help prevent aches. Carry your cushion from chair to chair. They are also excellent in the car.

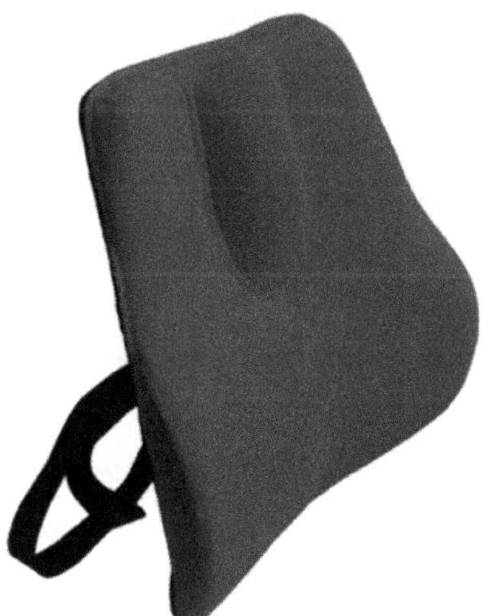

Self-Hypnosis Tapes

Because such a lot of the way your body responds to trauma and healing is controlled by your mind, I wanted to put mine in the best frame possible. I listened to audios specifically designed for assisting with good health, healing, and for boosting the immune system. There are a small number on the market but I used "*Pain Control Collection*" from the Personal Enhancement Series by Darren Stephens available from www.HypnosisCollection.com. I simply put in my earphones as I was going to sleep at night.

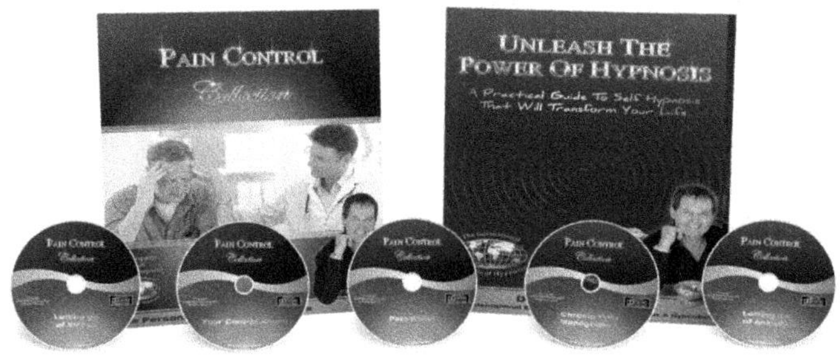

Pillows Again

Once home in your own bed the use of pillow or a body pillow is much easier with more room to get them in to the positions that best support your particular sore spots. I found a pillow between my knees a great relief for the drag on my back and a pillow at my tummy soft and supportive against my wound. Play with them until you find what gives you relief.

More Physio

You may remember my advice for physio in hospital was DO IT. The same applies at home. It's likely you'll be sent home with an exercise program from the hospital rehabilitation team – follow the program! If you're not given anything from the hospital make the effort to find a physio who has worked with people who have had your type of surgery. Don't be afraid to ring around and ask the question so you don't waste your time, and theirs, by going to a clinic that has no experience with your particular surgery.

While some exercises are universal, there are specific exercises for anterior v posterior surgery, for upper back v lumbar surgery. Ask the question, find a physio that suits, and then follow whatever program they devise for you. Also remember that if a particular exercise causes you pain, stop doing it until you can discuss it with the therapist. Otherwise, exercise your way to good health.

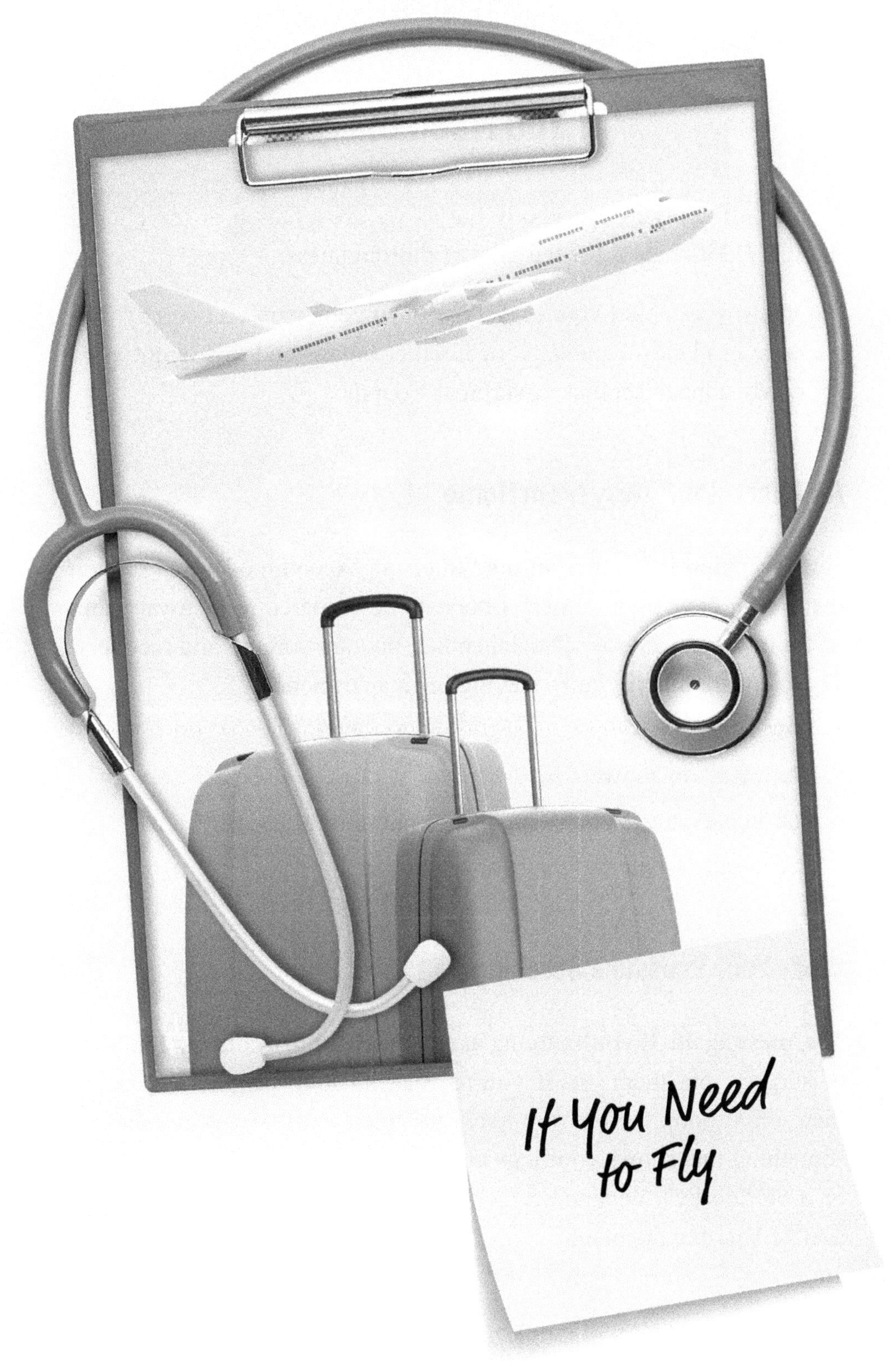
If You Need
to Fly

If You Need to Fly

This won't apply to everybody but as we are a nation of travellers I thought I'd include it for the sake of thoroughness.

For a few weeks after your surgery your surgeon won't let you fly. The pressure in planes expands your internal organs and this is not good for newly adjusted spines or surgical wounds.

An Apartment Away from Home

Just recapping in brief from the "Interstate Accommodation" section that if you have your surgery interstate be prepared to be away from home for two to four weeks, depending on your surgery and recovery. Try to ensure that if you're staying in an apartment it:

- is self contained.
- has a walk in shower.
- has an elevator if you're on the second floor or above.
- is centrally located to the shops

Wear Your Pressure Stockings

Yes, these again. If you're flying at any time within a couple of months of surgery, put them on. If you're wearing long pants you can put them on at home before you leave for the airport. If you're wearing something that shows your legs and don't want to look like an invalid or a bit "dorky", depending on your perspective, put them on once you've boarded the plane.

Book a Flexible Fare

Yes, I know it costs more, but you've had surgery and sometimes your plans have to change. Your surgeon may think you're not fit to fly, you may have complications after surgery, you might suffer a setback, or just not feel up to it. Rather than having to argue with the airline or pay penalties and flight differences it's much easier to have purchased a flight you can easily move.

A Medical Clearance to Fly

I discovered this one by accident, and lucky I did! Airlines won't let you fly for up to twelve weeks after back surgery unless you have a specific written medical clearance from your surgeon. You obtain the form by ringing your airline.

Now, if the airline doesn't know you've had surgery then most people don't bother with the form – right or wrong, that's just the truth of it. Be warned that if they suspect, you let it slip, someone tells them, they ask about the metal in your back setting off the screening detectors, or for a variety of other reasons they come to know you've had surgery, they are obliged to deny you access to the flight unless you have a medical clearance.

I think it's easier to get it signed by your surgeon at your post op visit and get it to cover the whole twelve-week period so you don't need to go back to them if you need to fly more than once.

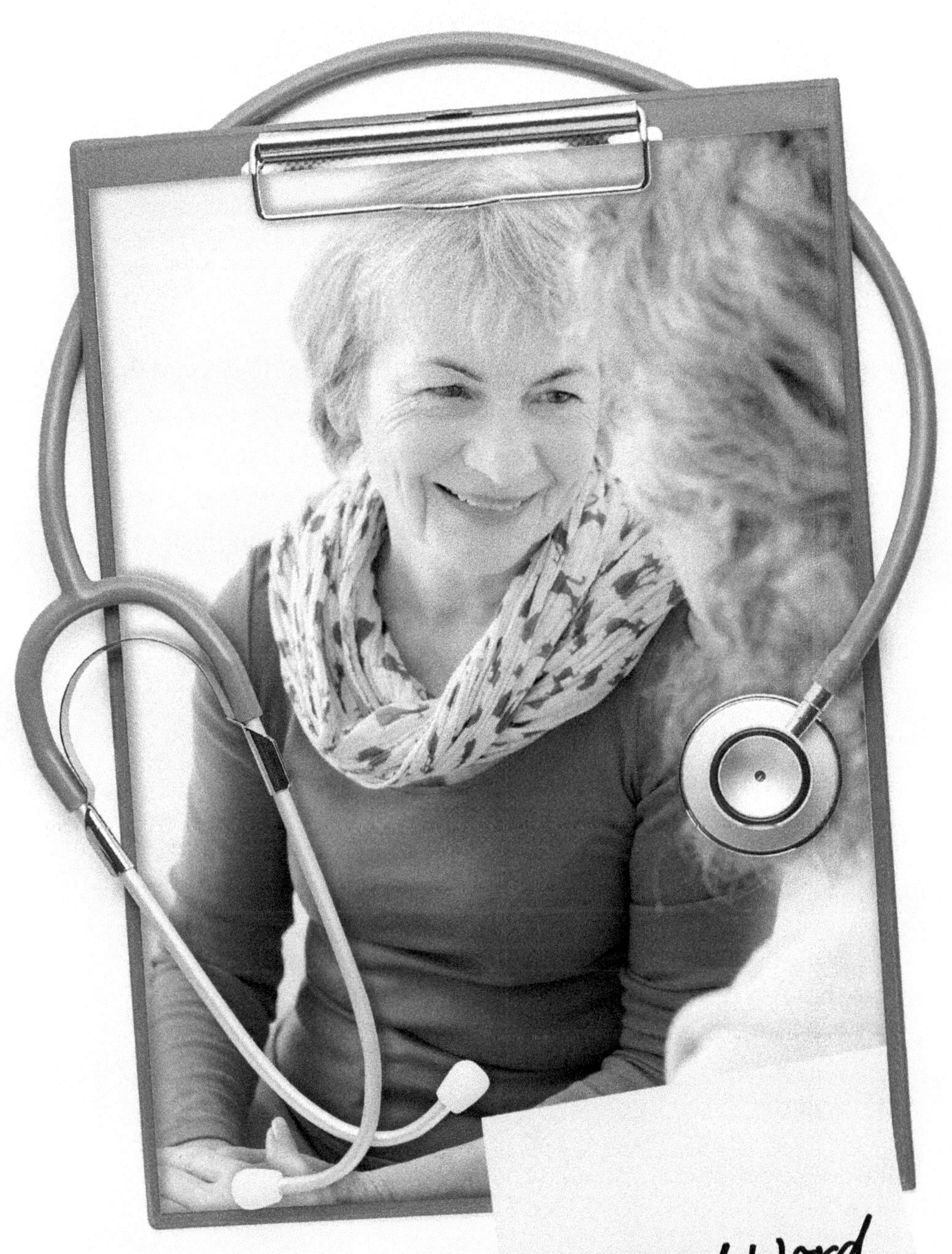

A Final Word

A Final Word

The first couple of weeks after surgery can sometimes be a little tougher than you are expecting.

Try to remember it's such a short period of time in the scheme of things. You may have had your back problems for years or even decades; a few weeks is nothing! The back pain you experienced previously served no purpose other than to alert you to the fact that something was wrong. Often it may have felt like there was no end in sight.

After surgery most people experience an immediate reduction in their old pain. Also the back pain you may feel now is a healing pain. You are on your way to getting better. Celebrate this! Know that what you have is short term and every day brings you closer to your goal of great health and a pain free life.

I hope this book has given you a little bit of clarity, some idea of what to expect, and some useful tips (from those who have been there and used them) to help make those first few weeks easier.

Know that my best wishes and thoughts are with you. Go, good luck, and get on with your new life.

Warm regards

Jackie

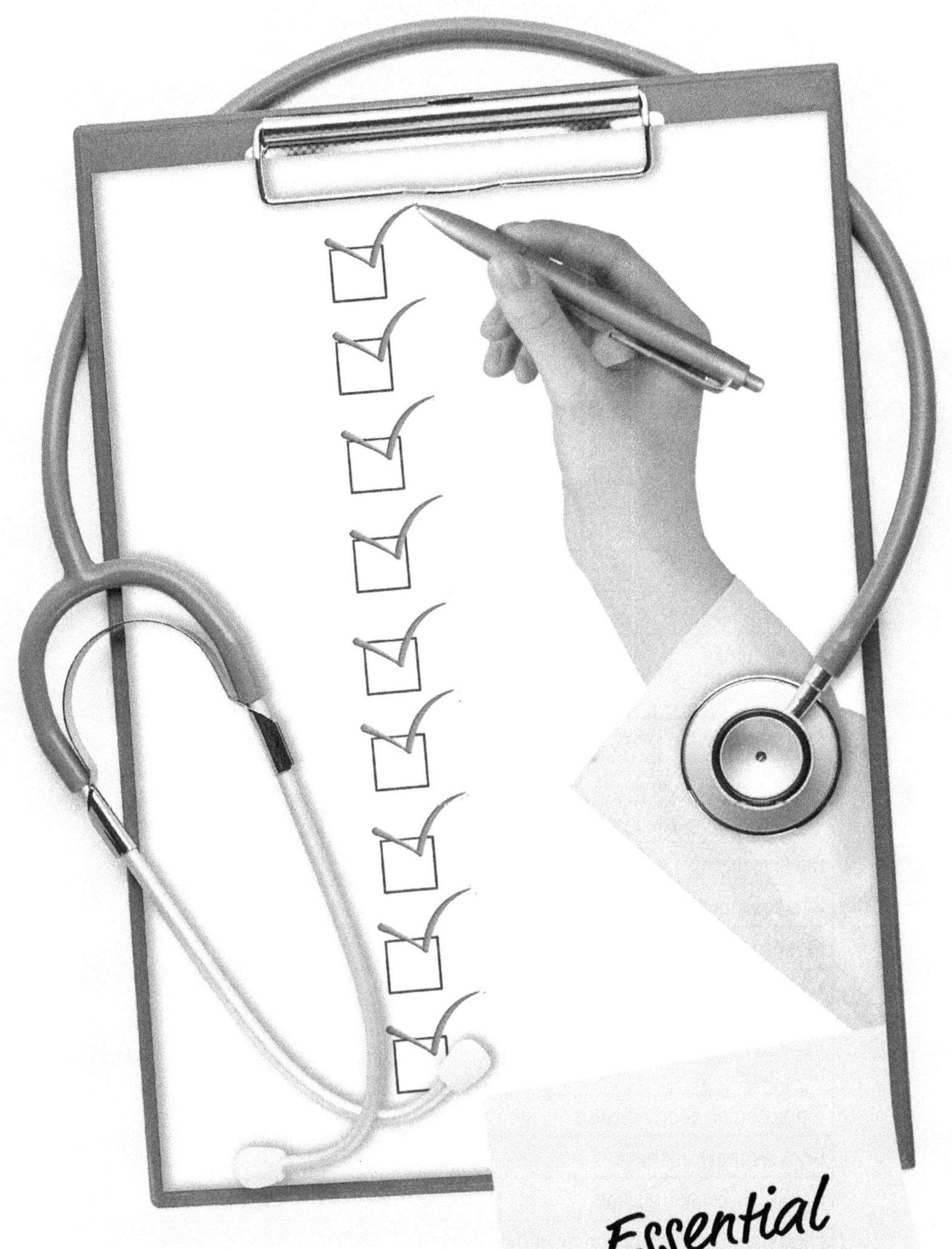
Essential
Checklists

Essential Checklists

The following two lists are guides only. Cross off anything not relevant to you and add anything that you think of that you particularly want or need.

Shopping List (What to buy before I go in to Hospital)

Item	Purchased ✔
Body pillow	
Books	
Magazines	
Puzzle books	
Sharpie pens	
Pyjamas	
Loose comfortable underwear	
Prescription medication	
Barley sugar	
Glasses chain	
Plastic stool	
Four pronged cane	
Long handled pinchers	
Sick bags	
Sippy cup or bendy straws	
Back support cushion	
Healing hypnosis audios	
Long handled body brush or body sponge	

Taking to Hospital List

Item	Packed ✔
Books	
Magazines	
Puzzle books	
Sharpie pens	
Pyjamas	
Slip on shoes or slippers	
Loose comfortable underwear	
Prescription medication	
Bowel medication	
Glasses chain	
Healing hypnosis audios	
Toiletries bag (fully stocked)	
Face washer (or two)	
Barley sugar	
Protein snacks / Other snacks	
Loose going home clothes	
Mobile phone and charger	
Ipad	

About the Author

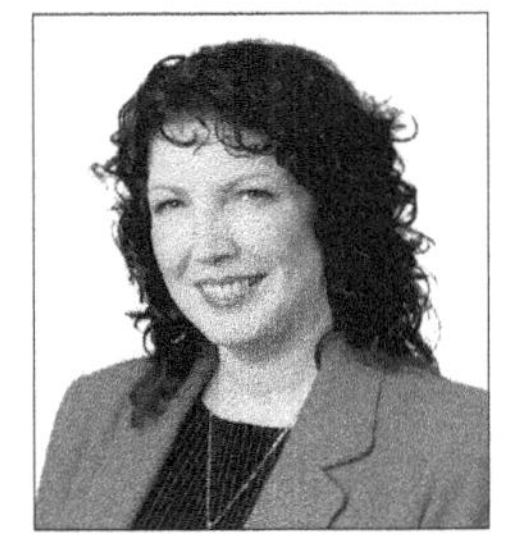

Jackie is an author, consultant, businesswoman, mother and, above all else, an educator. Her careers have been many and varied, ranging from corporate to small business, teaching to university lecturing, consulting, coaching and public speaking.

Jackie's appearance on many television programs, and the plethora of articles published about, and by, her in magazines and newspapers has ensured she is a sought after consultant and speaker on the international stage.

Her knowledge, and mastery, of techniques for improving and utilising the best available mindset has allowed her to travel the world speaking to individuals, corporations and groups. Regardless of her audience, be it a one on one with a world leader or a stage presentation to over 5000, Jackie's ability to take the complex and make it simple and understandable is what endears her to people.

She carefully blends her career demands with her most important role as a parent. She spends her time living between Melbourne and Queensland with her husband Darren and their seven children.

www.TipsForBackSurgery.com

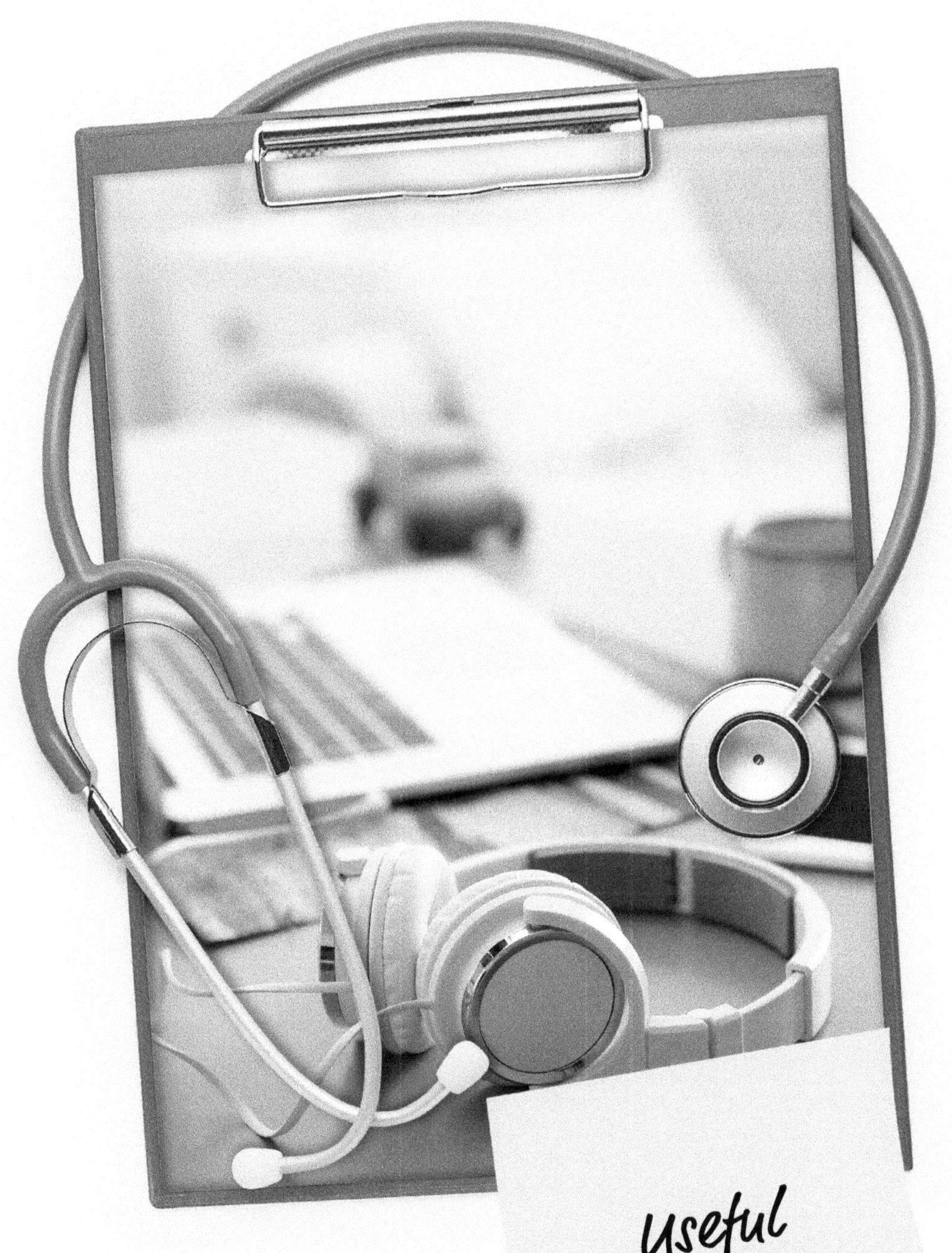

Useful Resources

Useful Resources

Healing Self Hypnosis Packs
Available from www.HypnosisCollection.com
or Global Publishing Group on +61 3 9739 4686.

Three that may be useful in this context are: *Pain Control Collection*, *Overnight Weight Loss*, and *How To Stop Smoking*.

Dr Matthew Scott Young
Gold Coast, Queensland, Australia.
Phone: +61 7 5528 06477
Email: info@goldcoastspine.com.au

PhysioSpine
Gold Coast, Queensland, Australia.
Phone: +61 7 5635 7333
Email: reception@physiospine.com

Some of the other products mentioned are available online or at large pharmacies (usually independent rather than discount chains).

Pain Control Collection

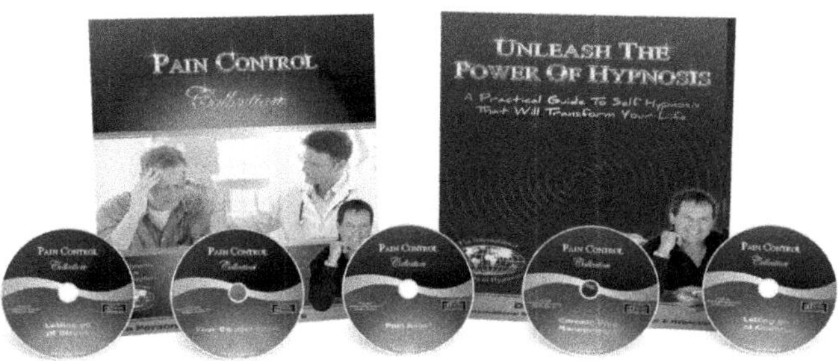

Although pain is an important signal from the body that something needs attention, and no unusual pain should just be ignored, it is useful to remember that the experience of pain always includes a psychological component.

And that means that you can influence the experience of pain.

The **Pain Control Hypnosis Collection** from the ***Darren Stephens Personal Enhancement Series*** was designed to help you battle pain. Whether you are healing after an operation or injury, or whether you are dealing with chronic illness or disability, or even if you just have a headache, the techniques contained in this program will stand you in good stead.

This collection includes these 5 tracks essential for controlling pain:

- **Letting Go of Stress** is an essential tool which will empower your sense of autonomy and control and allow you to relax and sleep peacefully
- **Your Control Panel** gives you the key to success for, and the ultimate control system to enhance, every function of your mind and body including your pain centres
- **Letting Go of Anxiety** will help to ensure you stay calm in stressful situations and teach you to stop assuming the worst which exacerbates painful symptoms
- **Pain Relief** has been put together specifically to help you modify, dull or remove the experience of pain
- **Chronic Pain Management** will empower anyone suffering from chronic conditions to significantly affect the levels of pain that they encounter

www.HypnosisCollection.com

Overnight Weight Loss Collection

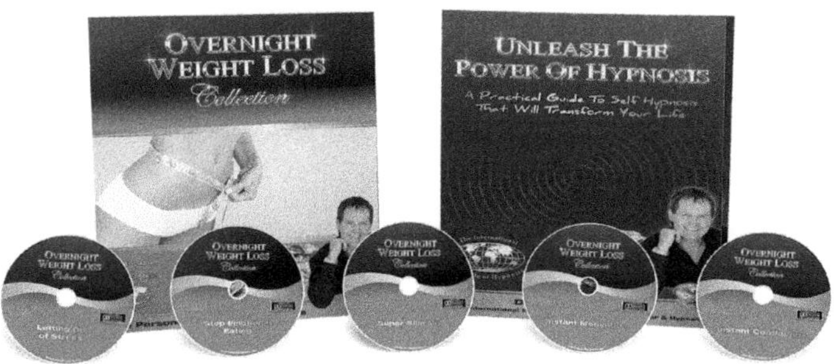

Starting a diet is easy, as everyone knows. People do it every day. And often the first surge of enthusiasm can give you a real high, and keep you going for a short while. But it's all too common for people to experience a falling off of their motivation after a while. This can happen for many reasons, but once it has happened, it can feel so much easier to just go back to the old unhealthy ways – until you're ready to start a new diet. And then it starts all over again...

The **Overnight Weight Loss Hypnosis Collection** from the ***Darren Stephens Personal Enhancement Series*** was developed to help people who want to escape from the trap of yo-yo dieting, and find a way to get their excess weight off and keep it off, that will actually work and that they can stick to.

This collection includes these 5 essential tracks for anyone wanting to lose weight:

- **Instant Motivation** will excite your unconscious into action and give you the motivation to keep going and keep challenging yourself to lose those extra kilos
- **Instant Confidence** will re-inforce your self belief and give you the strength to tackle situations that would usually have you reaching for comfort food with ease
- **Super Slim Me** will give you an effective method for developing – and keeping – the instinctive behaviour patterns and mindset of a naturally healthy and fit person
- **Letting Go of Stress** is an essential tool which will empower your sense of autonomy and control and allow you to relax and enjoy life as you lose weight and gain fitness
- **Stop Emotional Eating** will retrain your brain to stop feeding your emotions with food instead of with appropriate action

www.HypnosisCollection.com

How to Quit Smoking Collection

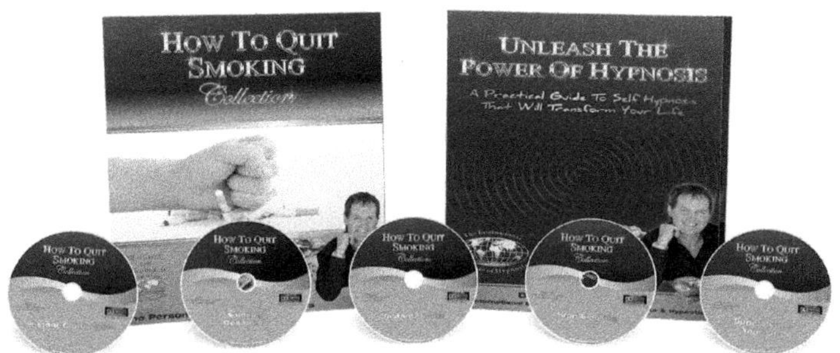

This How to Quit Smoking Hypnosis Collection has a unique approach to helping people who no longer want to smoke. Why? Because this is not a how to stop smoking programme.

It is a how to become a non-smoker program - and a non-smoker is someone for whom smoking is just not relevant.

The **How to Quit Smoking Hypnosis Collection** from the ***Darren Stephens Personal Enhancement Series*** was developed to help you escape from the smoking trap and live the healthy and in control life you want to live.

This collection includes these 5 tracks essential for anyone seeking to become a non-smoker:

- **Supercharge Your Life** will help you develop the mental and emotional skills essential for you to quit smoking
- **Instant Confidence** focuses on providing you with the confidence to handle any situation, any time, with anyone without a cigarette
- **Instant Health** will re-inforce your self belief and give you the strength to tackle this challenge, push yourself harder and face difficult situations without cravings
- **Stop Smoking** provides you with all the psychological tools you need to kick the nicotine habit
- **Smoking Cessation** will empower you with all the tools you need to become a non-smoker for good

www.HypnosisCollection.com

Instant Health & Fitness Collection

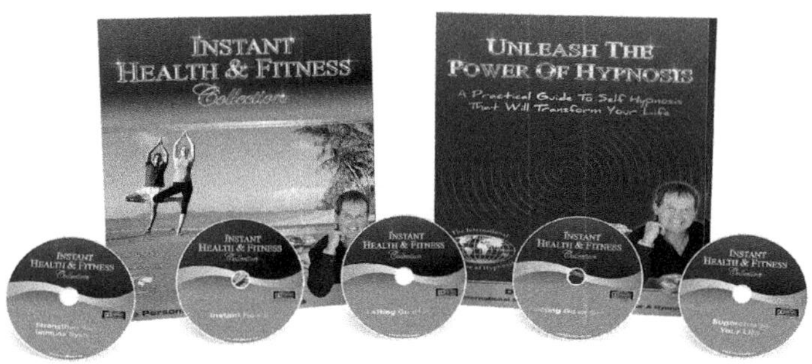

How do you keep yourself committed to your ongoing health and fitness when the glow of your New Year resolutions has passed? How do you really get started (and keep going) when you know that you need to exercise, and eat better and more mindfully, if you want to stay fit and healthy?

There are a million diet and exercise regimes out there but do any of them really have the answer?

The **Instant Health and Fitness Hypnosis Collection** from the ***Darren Stephens Personal Enhancement Series*** was developed to provide an effective, powerful and easy way for people to inspire themselves to take up and stick to a healthier, more active life.

This collection includes these 5 essential tracks for a healthy lifestyle:

- **Supercharge Your Life** will help you develop the mental and emotional skills essential for you to reach your peak in all areas of your life
- **Letting Go of Fear** provides an effective and powerful way for you to take back command of your emotional responses
- **Letting Go of Stress** is a liberating and empowering experience which gives you a greater sense of autonomy and control
- **Instant Health** will re-inforce the importance of and inspire you to live a more healthy and active life
- **Strengthen Your Immune System** is a powerful tool designed to enhance the functioning of your immune system

www.HypnosisCollection.com

www.ingramcontent.com/pod-product-compliance
Ingram Content Group UK Ltd.
Pitfield, Milton Keynes, MK11 3LW, UK
UKHW020139250726
13967UKWH00002B/743

9 781925 288391